LIVING WITH DEMENTIA

LIVING WITH DEMENTIA

RELATIONS, RESPONSES AND AGENCY IN EVERYDAY LIFE

Edited by
LARS-CHRISTER HYDÉN AND
ELEONOR ANTELIUS

 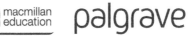

First published 2017 by
PALGRAVE

Palgrave in the UK is an imprint of Macmillan Publishers Limited,
registered in England, company number 785998, of 4 Crinan Street,
London, N1 9XW.

Palgrave® and Macmillan® are registered trademarks in the United States,
the United Kingdom, Europe and other countries.

ISBN: 978–1–137–59374–0 paperback

This book is printed on paper suitable for recycling and made from fully
managed and sustained forest sources. Logging, pulping and manufacturing
processes are expected to conform to the environmental regulations of the
country of origin.

A catalogue record for this book is available from the British Library.

A catalog record for this book is available from the Library of Congress.

CONTENTS

NOTES ON THE CONTRIBUTORS

Eleonor Antelius is a medical anthropologist who received her PhD in Health and Society, and currently holds a position as Senior Lecturer at the division of Aging and Later Life at Linköping University, Sweden, and as Assistant Director of the Center for Dementia Research (CEDER). Her research primarily concerns communicative disorders in relation to meaning-making processes and being able to maintain and uphold a sense of self. Social interaction, identity, embodiment, ethnicity and cross-cultural perceptions and experiences of illnesses and aging are all central concepts in her research. She has initiated and coordinates the international research network *Different Dementias* and she is elected president of the *Nordic Research Network on Ethnicity and Dementia*.

Ruth Bartlett is an Associate Professor at the Faculty of Health Sciences, University of Southampton, UK. She gained a PhD in Sociology and has a BA in Politics and MA in Cultural Politics. She has a special interest in care and citizenship in relation to people with dementia, and participatory research, including diary methods. Ruth is Director of the Faculty's Doctoral Training Centre in Dementia Care and Programme Lead for MSc Complex Care in Older People.

Anna Ekström holds a position as Postdoc at the Center for Dementia Research (CEDER) and her work focuses on interaction and collaboration in activities that involve people with dementia. Using video documentation of how couples living together interact and collaborate around everyday household activities, questions related to agency, participation and distribution of knowledge and competences are investigated and discussed. The studies are conducted within an ethnomethodological tradition where social practices are taken as the primary research object.

Ingrid Hellström has a position as Associate Professor at the Department of Social and Welfare Studies and Researcher at the Center for Dementia Research at Linköping University, Sweden. She has a background in clinical gerontological nursing, especially in the care of persons living with dementia. Her main research interest is people living with dementia and their families in different stages of the disease.

Lars-Christer Hydén received his PhD in Psychology from Stockholm University, Sweden. His current position is as Full Professor of Social Psychology at

Linköping University, Sweden, and as Director of the Center for Dementia Research (CEDER). His research primarily concerns how people with Alzheimer's disease and their significant others interact and use language – especially narrative – as a way to sustain and negotiate identity and a sense of self. He has published articles in international journals and edited books about narrative research, for instance *Health, Culture and Illness: Broken Narratives* (together with Jens Brockmeier, Routledge 2008) and *Beyond Loss: Dementia, Identity, Personhood* (together with Hilde Lindemann & Jens Brockmeier, Oxford University Press 2014), as well as the monograph *Entangled Narratives. Collaborative Storytelling and the Re-Imagining of Dementia.*

Danielle Jones, Danielle Jones holds a PhD in Sociology from the University of York, and is currently a Lecturer in Dementia Studies at the School of Dementia Studies, Bradford University, UK. Her research interests include the experience of living with dementia, with a particular focus on relationships in families in which a member has dementia, and the use of Conversation Analysis for developing memory assessment and diagnostic procedures. Danielle is the founder of the Dementia Communication Research Network (DCRN), an international network of scholars involved in undertaking research on dementia and communication.

Lisa Folkmarson Käll is Associate Senior Lecturer in Gender Studies at Stockholm University and Research Associate in Philosophy of Medicine and Medical Ethics at the Center for Dementia Research, Linköping University, Sweden. She holds a PhD in Women's Studies from Clark University, USA and a PhD in Philosophy from the Center for Subjectivity Research, University of Copenhagen, Denmark. Her work is in the area of contemporary continental philosophy and feminist philosophy, focusing on questions concerning embodied subjectivity, intersubjectivity, vulnerability and the relation between selfhood and otherness. She is currently working on a project on conceptualizations of subjectivity in relation to age-related dementia. Käll is editor of *Bodies, Boundaries and Vulnerabilities: Interrogating Social, Cultural and Political Aspects of Embodiment* (Springer 2015) and *Dimensions of Pain* (Routledge 2013) and co-editor of *Feminist Phenomenology and Medicine* (SUNY Press 2014).

Camilla Lindholm is an Acting Professor in Scandinavian languages at Helsinki University, Finland. Her main research areas are interaction in institutional settings, asymmetric interaction involving participants with communication impairment and structures in spoken Swedish. Lindholm takes an interest in applying her research findings and creating a dialogue with society.

Ali Reza Majlesi, a collaborator with the Center for Dementia Research at Linköping University, Sweden, is an interaction analyst. He has conducted his postdoctoral research on communication and joint activities with people with dementia. His research interests lie in methods and practices including the mobilization of embodied resources, in interaction with people with various communicative and cognitive abilities. Majlesi is currently affiliated with Stockholm University as a Senior Lecturer in the Department of Education.

Ann-Charlotte Nedlund, is a Senior Lecturer of Politics and Policy Analysis in Aging and Later Life at Division Ageing and Social Change (ASC) and CEDER (Centre for Dementia Research), Department of Social and Welfare Studies at Linköping University, Sweden. She is also working at the National Centre for Setting Priorities in Healthcare and Medical Education: Interprofessional Learning, both at Linköping University. She has initiated and is a coordinator of the International Research Network on Citizenship and Dementia. Her research primarily concerns issues related to health and social policy, citizenship, legitimacy, democracy and the welfare system, and further, how the conditions for citizens with dementia to practise their citizenship are regarded and realised.

Linda Örulv, PhD in Health and Society, currently holds a position as a Junior Fellow Researcher at NISAL – National Institute for the Study of Ageing and Later Life. Her main research focus is meaning-making and identity work in situations where such things are brought to a head or somehow challenged, as is the case with Alzheimer's disease and other age-related progressive dementia disorders. She has a special interest in narrating as a way to make sense of the world and to maintain one's self-identity in interaction with others and in her latest studies she has, for more than six years, followed a self-help group for people with dementia, primarily focusing upon interaction and conversations within the group, but also upon how citizens with dementia organise themselves.

Elizabeth Peel is a Professor of Communication and Social Interaction and Director of Research, Department of Social Sciences, Loughborough University, and a Fellow of the British Psychological Society. She is a critical social psychologist with interests in gender, sexualities and chronic illness. Her current research centres on communication and conversation in dementia care.

Charlotta Plejert is an Associate Professor of Linguistics at the Department of Culture and Communication, Linköping University, Sweden. Her main research interests are language and interaction involving people with communicative impairments, multilingualism and ethnicity in dementia, and language acquisition over the lifespan. She is co-editor of *Journal of Interactional Research in Communication Disorders* (equinox).

Parvin Pooremamali is a registered occupational therapist and currently holds a position as Assistant Researcher at Lund University, Sweden. Her dissertation *Culture, occupation and occupational therapy in a mental health care context: the* *challenges of meeting the needs of Middle Eastern immigrants* concerns the need for culturally adapted occupational therapy as well as adapted care and rehabilitation within psychiatric care. Parvin's research mainly concerns activity and participation as well as meaning making and well-being among people with ethnoculturally diverse backgrounds.

Christina Samuelsson received her PhD in Speech and Language Pathology from Lund University, Sweden, in 2004. Her current position is Associate Professor of Speech and Language Pathology at Linköping University, Sweden. Her research mainly concerns how people with communicative disabilities such as developmental language disorders, aphasia and dementia interact and use language, with a specific focus on prosody.

Annika Taghizadeh Larsson is a Senior Lecturer at the National Institute for the Study of Ageing and Later Life (NISAL) at Linköping University, Sweden. Her research interests mainly comprise questions and issues at the intersection of social gerontology and disability studies, including social policy and welfare for older people with disabilities and aging with early-onset impairments.

1

INTRODUCTION: FROM EMPTY VESSELS TO ACTIVE AGENTS

Lars-Christer Hydén and Eleonor Antelius

The aim of this introductory chapter is to present a background to the emerging field of dementia studies and thus also to the chapters in this book and its primary agenda: to offer an alternative to the common care perspective on dementia and instead present a focus on everyday life with dementia and what people living with dementia in fact can accomplish together with other persons. We begin with just a few words about the definition of dementia and some basic epidemiological facts.

Epidemiology

Dementia is not *one* disease, but an overall term describing a broad spectrum of symptoms, which can be caused by a multitude of diseases and injuries to the brain (see Hughes, 2011). As such, dementia is a syndrome – and can be of both chronic and progressive nature – in which there is deterioration in cognitive function beyond what might be expected from normal aging (World Health Organization, *Dementia*). Mainly, the dementias are divided into three subcategories:

1 *Primary degenerative diseases*: In these diseases, dementia is caused by an abnormal extent of unnatural degeneration of brain cells. Typical of these diseases is that one cannot tell when it starts; they are insidious and the person with dementia will experience a gradual deterioration.

2 *Vascular dementias*: These diseases are caused by cutting off of the oxygen supply to the brain (usually by blood clots or strokes); symptoms are often sudden and noticeable.

3 *Secondary diseases*: These are diseases and injuries that *could*, but need not, lead to dementia. All in all, more than 80 diseases and types of injuries could cause dementia symptoms, for instance brain tumours, alcohol abuse or traumatic brain injuries.

Most of the chapters in this volume are concerned with age-related dementias, that is, the first subcategory of primary degenerative diseases. However, the discussions and arguments presented in the chapters are in no way specific to these types of dementias; living with dementia and the understanding of persons with dementia as active agents are relevant to all types of dementias even though symptoms can be extremely varied. The reason the chapters revolve (mainly) around age-related dementias is due to the fact that they are, by far, the most common of the dementias.

Alzheimer's disease, one type of primary degenerative dementia, accounts for 60–70% of all cases of dementia, and the World Health Organization (WHO) estimates that the number of people living with (all sorts of) dementias worldwide currently is 47.5 million, a number increasing by 7.7 million each year and projected to reach 75.6 million by 2030 and almost triple by 2050 to reach 135.5 million people (WHO, 2016). The number of people living with dementia is expected to continue to rise as people, in both industrialized and developing countries, tend to live longer and longer, and as such have a higher risk of developing an age-related dementia disease such as Alzheimer's disease. The rates of increase are, however, not uniform; much of this increase is attributed to rising numbers of people living with dementia in low- and middle-income countries (WHO, 2016). A study of prevalence estimates for every WHO world region forecasts that in developed (high-income) countries there will be an increase of 100% between the years 2001 and 2040, while in India, China, South Asia and the Western Pacific, the increase will more likely be 300% (Ferri et al., 2005).

One major concern that these increasing numbers have sparked is the social and economic impacts of the dementias in terms of medical costs, direct social costs and cost of informal care. And although such numbers can be quite intimidating (in 2010, the total global societal costs of dementia were estimated to be US$ 604 billion, corresponding to 1.0% of the worldwide gross domestic product, WHO, 2016) the mere fact that almost 135.5 million people worldwide will be living with dementia by the year 2050 is evidence for considering the more human aspects and tangible effects of *living with dementia*.

Dementia studies

By tradition dementia has been defined primarily in terms of loss: loss of cognitive and communicative competencies, loss of identity and personhood and loss of personal relations. Persons with dementia have been portrayed as increasingly dependent on others, in particular in terms of being care receivers while their significant others have been seen more as caregivers than as spouses, children or relatives. However, during the last two decades this view has been challenged, especially by pointing out that persons with dementia do not become empty vessels, devoid of cognitive, emotional and communicative competencies. Instead, a focus on remaining abilities has started to prevail.

Much of the medical and psychological research about dementia has been organized around attempts to describe the neurodegenerative brain processes involved in the various forms of dementia. Research in the care sciences has mainly focused on providing knowledge about how care can best be provided for persons with dementia and which care interventions are beneficial. Not seldom the focus has been on the relatives and how they can best cope with caring for a person with a disease such as dementia. At the same time, a new field of research about persons with dementia has emerged – *dementia studies* – involving researchers with a background in areas like anthropology, language, sociology, philosophy and other human and social sciences. Central to dementia studies is to approach persons with dementia as active agents, in their own lives as well as in their local communities as residents. This agency-based approach to dementia studies has actualized a number of issues, some of which are discussed in this book. We have focused on a number of issues that involve a shift in the way persons with dementia are defined and described. In the following, four such issues will be discussed.

Context: from care to a life with dementia

The fact that dementia primarily has been seen as a disease has to do with the context in which the patient with dementia has been encountered and described – namely primarily in care settings. Hence it has been natural to define dementia primarily in medical terms and describe the consequences in terms of losses of abilities. As no real treatment for dementia is available, support has mainly been formulated in terms of care delivered by care professionals (nurses, occupational therapists, etc.).

Not least for demographic reasons, people with dementia are much more visible in today's society compared with the situation some 50 years ago: people live longer and thus more people will get a dementia diagnosis. People with dementia predominantly continue to live at home for many years and will spend only the final years in some form of residential-care facility. Living at home, persons diagnosed with dementia will live with their spouses and families and in their local communities.

This fact is a strong reason behind the shift in the field of dementia studies towards an interest in the experience of *living with dementia*, that is, the experience of being a person living with dementia in various everyday contexts: at home in their local community, together with spouses, family, friends and neighbours. At the end of the life of the person with dementia, the everyday context shifts to a care context, inhabited by other persons with dementia and professional care staff.

Point of view – perspectives

There has been a shift in focus from primarily studying loss of various functions to studying people with dementia as active agents using their remaining abilities to sustain and change their own lives in relation to the progressing disease. This involves re-negotiating the organization of everyday life as well as identity and relations with other persons, from family members to friends and neighbours. This shift also involves perspectives. Perspective has to do with the point of view not only of other persons but also the world. In philosophy, linguistics and literary studies, a first-person perspective means taking the perspective of the experiencing person; a second-person perspective is the perspective of the participants engaged in acting, focusing on other persons or the surrounding world; finally, the third-person perspective is the spectator perspective: seeing and describing other persons without engaging with them.

In the field of dementia studies we can witness a clear shift from a preference for a spectator (third-person perspective) to an interest in the experience (first-person perspective) of the person with dementia, to seeing the person with dementia as engaged in interaction with others (second-person perspective).

What is typical of what often is called the medical perspective on dementia and the person with dementia is the *third-person – spectator – perspective*. That is, the disease and the consequences are described by clinicians, researchers and care staff as something happening and belonging to another person. In texts, this can often be seen in the use of pronouns: the person living with dementia is often depicted as a 'he' or 'she' and the disease is an 'it'; that is, both the person with illness and the illness are described as something 'out there' by someone who is not ill.

A problem with this perspective is that it often does not allow much knowledge about how the ill person experiences the illness – something that often is important in order to support or help the person with illness. The voice of the person with dementia is represented, selected and edited by the other. These constraints have resulted in a shift towards an interest in a *first-person perspective* on dementia, that is, an interest in how people living with dementia actually describe and experience themselves, their lives and relations as well as their position in the community. A focus on a first-person perspective is an attempt to give persons with dementia a possibility to voice their own experiences. The possibilities of a first-person perspective of a person living with dementia have been questioned because persons with dementia often are challenged in terms of using their communicative resources. Although this might be true, it also is true that persons with dementia often are believed to have fewer abilities than they actually have. Already in 1993, the researchers and social workers Victoria Cottrell and Richard Schulz wrote about listening to the voice of persons with dementia:

In part because cognitive deficits lie at the core of AD, researchers have assumed that data collected from demented individuals (sic!) is inherently unreliable and therefore not useful. This narrow view ignores the variability in the communicative abilities of individuals with dementia and reflects a very limited perspective on research methods that might be used to ascertain their views. (Cottrell & Schulz, 1993, p. 210)

Further, it could be pointed out that involving persons with dementia in telling about their lives is about being involved as listener in joint attempts to make meaning and communication. Although it might be the case that this process sometimes is more elaborate and time-consuming compared to talking to so-called healthy persons, it is not an argument for abstaining from becoming involved with people living with dementia – rather, it is an argument about allocating more time.

Through and through, the first-person perspective has also been supplemented by what often is called a second-person perspective, that is, trying to find out how persons with dementia interact with other persons (with or without dementia). In engaging in interaction, persons approach and address each other as 'thou'; they do not describe the other, but rather ask questions, request things or tell about their experiences in a way so the other person not only can understand but also can respond. Understanding people with dementia from a second-person perspective implies an understanding of the ways persons are engaged – emotionally as well as cognitively and linguistically – with each other and with the world (see Schilbach et al., 2013). A typical example would be persons engaged in a conversation: they direct their attention to each other, taking in not only the words spoken but also each other's gazes, body postures and gestures; and they adjust their own words and non-verbal signs in order to make the right impression on the other.

Understanding how interaction is organized in, for instance, conversations involving persons with dementia will help to understand how the person with dementia collaborates with his or her conversational partner in order to create a shared understanding of what they are talking about. In conversations involving persons with dementia – as in all conversations – this involves understanding the ways the participants together repair and keep the conversation going in the face of the challenges the person with dementia encounters.

Both the first-person perspective and the second-person perspective are important tools for developing knowledge about how persons with dementia and their spouses organize and re-organize their shared lives and how they deal with communicative challenges and challenges to their shared identities and further, how they make use of their communities, what facilitates them to use it and move around and what constrains and limits them from using it. What are the experiences of people with dementia to join forces and voice their shared concerns and demands?

There is also a connection among knowledge, practical actions and perspectives. A spectator perspective often implies delivering ready-made packages to be used by persons with dementia or their carers. Knowledge about living with dementia from a first- or second-person perspective is often more about explorations and discoveries that can be turned into shared learning experiences: doing and learning are fused. By starting this kind of collective learning process, individuals and local communities are better prepared to engage in interaction with persons living with dementia. This will have long-term positive and facilitating effects in the community.

From individuals to persons in collaboration

Many theories about citizenship, identity, autonomy, etc. rest on the notion of an individual equipped with fully functional cognitive and linguistic abilities (the emotional abilities are rarely discussed), able to speak, make decisions and act rationally. For instance, this is the case in political theory, in which the citizen is pictured as being able to take in and consider information and to take part in political activities and discussions. In psychological theory, the individual is supposed to be able to remember and communicate experiences on her own, and identities and selves belong to the individual. In ethical theory, individuals are the ones who consider situations involving choice and make decisions based on rational thinking.

The problem, of course, is that this individualistic focus does not work when it comes to understanding persons living with dementia. Persons with dementia do not fare well in those clinical or experimental settings constructed to evaluate a lone individual's abilities nor if voting behaviour is taken as the paradigmatic case for political activity. Persons with dementia challenge this kind of assumption, forcing human and social scientists to reconsider if the individual is the naturally given starting point. Research and practical experience have shown that persons with dementia often are much more capable if they engage in collaborative activities with other persons. The reason for this is that other people not only can support the person with dementia emotionally, but they can also share their cognitive and linguistic abilities with the person with dementia when they pursue a shared activity like preparing dinner. People doing things together is thus a better starting point for understanding what persons with dementia can or cannot do.

Methodological challenges

The understanding of persons with dementia as agents also implies research designs and research methods that are inclusive. For instance, traditionally persons with dementia have often been excluded from interview studies because they were considered impossible to interview. Including persons with dementia in research implies that a number of classical methods – from ethnographic observations and recordings to interviews – can be used, although they must be adapted to people with alternative cognitive and linguistic abilities.

Overview of the chapters

In Chapter 2 the philosopher Lisa Käll maps out different conceptualizations of subjectivity and selfhood that often are taken for granted as points of departure for predominant understandings of dementia diseases, for instance Alzheimer's disease. A common and well-established view of dementia, and perhaps especially of Alzheimer's disease, is that it will lead to a gradual disappearance of the person, leaving the body behind as an empty shell. Such an understanding rests on a strictly dualistic conception of the human being in terms of an inner mind and an outer body, where the inner mind is what constitutes a person's subjectivity and identity. The mind is furthermore often conceived exclusively in terms of cognition. Diminishment and loss of cognitive abilities are thus assumed to lead to a loss of subjectivity and to a death of the self, prior to the death of the body, in other words to what has often been referred to as 'social death'. Contesting this view of the person with dementia as disappearing and the victim of a mental and social death prior to actual death, much empirical research has demonstrated how cognitive and other capacities remain throughout the progression of the condition. While such a view has contributed to a significant improvement in our understanding of persons with conditions of dementia, it at the same time often rests on the same dualistic conception of the person, with the only difference that an inner mind is assumed to survive a diminishment of cognitive capacities. With the aim of clarifying conceptualizations of the subjectivity of dementia, this chapter will first discuss a traditional dualistic view of human subjectivity and then turn to attempts, primarily from phenomenological philosophy, at reconceptualising subjectivity beyond dualistic structures, taking into consideration its embodiment, relationality and situatedness.

In Chapter 3 the medical anthropologist Eleonor Antelius discusses cross-cultural perceptions of the dementias and how, in a world demarcated by growing migration, it is paramount to understand ethnocultural contextualization of dementia (and dementia care). By addressing how the dementias are experienced within a convergence of values, norms and traditions as well as individual and shared experiences, the chapter discusses how dementia needs to be de-medicalized in order to facilitate an extended analysis of dementia models in which social and cultural factors such as recognition of symptoms, help-seeking strategies, caregiving and coping become more apparent. By discussing the dementias as highly culturally demarcated and socially shaped, the chapter raises issues of transnational and migratory aspects of the dementias as well as highlighting the importance of never underestimating the impact cultural norms and traditions might play in regard to social interaction, care and care-seeking behaviours.

In Chapter 4 the political scientist Ann-Charlotte Nedlund and the sociologist Ruth Bartlett argue that the study of dementia policies could shed light on the possibilities for participation and decision-making as well as the various forms of formal support and their distribution. The use of a citizenship perspective in order to study and problematize situations for persons with dementia has received increasing attention during the last decade and, like other perspectives within dementia studies, it is signified by recognizing a person with dementia as an active agent with the right to be self-determinant, to formulate their own goals and to have power over their own lives. However, the definition and construction of citizenship and various categories and labels of citizens are seldom explicit, but often embedded in policies. Public policies are dynamic instruments where authorities, at various levels, give signals and legitimise how citizen groups are valued and regarded by other citizens, which attitudes and courses of action are regarded as appropriate and which services they can expect from welfare organisations, but also are instruments to change social constructions of citizenship and citizens. The policy process relates to the construction of political problems, whereas the construction of policy areas, targeted groups, goals and appropriate solutions does not begin until they are recognized as political problems. The process by which problems and their imminent solutions become recognized and thereby legitimate is a struggle over ideas, stories and interests in which various actors compete. Thus, the meaning of citizenship and the construction of citizens are constantly under negotiation and interpretation and therefore always undergoing change.

As citizenship always is constructed in intersecting social divisions, citizens and citizen groups will come to involve 'real' people who are differently situated in terms of gender, class, ethnicity, sexuality, ability, age, etc., where belonging to a specific policy target group will affect the distribution of rights, entitlements and obligations, that is, what the citizenship content will be. At the same time, policies and the construction of policy targets depend on which actors are involved in the policy process and, to be more specific, have the power to get involved or to be considered and on which actors claim or are claimed to have knowledge. Therefore, in order to be able to influence the content of citizenship, citizens need to have access to the policy processes. In this relation, policies have implications for citizenship and, in the long run, for democracy.

In Chapter 5 the linguists Charlotta Plejert, Daniella Jones and Elizabeth Peel describe and highlight pathways towards a dementia diagnosis, starting at the point when a person has been referred to a memory clinic for evaluation. A dementia diagnosis is often the end of a long process during which the person who receives the diagnosis might quite early on have discovered various troubles in everyday life; troubles that they initially tried to remedy, manage or ignore or perhaps even attempted to hide. Sometimes, relatives have also noticed these troubles. Contacting formal care (e.g. a health-care centre, and subsequently a memory clinic) due to the troubles experienced often implies a change of social status and identity and may affect the relations between, for instance, family members and friends. When a patient is referred to a memory clinic for evaluation, a fairly extensive and standardised procedure awaits. A dementia evaluation is complex and comprises different activities, such as history-taking (medical interview), formal tests of cognitive functioning, physical and psychiatric examinations, and ancillary investigations, blood tests, brain scans and lumbar punctures. For many patients and their relatives, this is an emotionally taxing experience. For people born abroad, who might speak another mother tongue, and might have limited educational background (i.e. literacy skills), going through a dementia evaluation may be even *more* challenging, as evaluations and appointments often are mediated by an interpreter, which, although primarily beneficial, makes tasks longer in duration and may affect the possibility for all nuances of the patient's experiences of their trouble to come forth. Despite an interpreter's professionalism, using one may also make it more difficult for patients and doctors to build trust and rapport during the evaluation. In addition, many tests of cognitive functioning that are used during neuropsychological evaluation are not adapted to patients with limited educational background and are not translated and validated in all languages needed, which makes this part of the evaluation particularly challenging for everyone involved. Because the chapter will discuss data from clinical evaluations of both native patients and ethnoculturally diverse patients, an ethnoculturally informed account will be provided.

In Chapter 6, speech therapist Christina Samuelsson and linguists Anna Ekström, Ali Reza Majlesi and Camilla Lindholm investigate the conjointly collaborative achievement of daily activities involving persons with dementia in home environments and the potential for persons with dementias to be active participants in daily activities. Because dementia affects a person's cognitive and communicative abilities and thereby also limits their means and opportunities to participate in everyday activities, persons with dementia often require assistance in taking part in and carrying out daily chores. As research in dementia studies extensively points out, while it is important for people with dementia to participate in social activities (to improve the quality of life for people with dementia), it is then often required that someone else both plan and monitor the activities. Hence, practices involved in activities that are conjointly accomplished through collaboration between people with dementia and their caregivers (usually spouses) are explored in this part of the book. This conjointly accomplished collaboration comprises both verbal and nonverbal interaction, and while the importance of collaboration has been underlined in other studies of dementia, much of the previous research on dementia and everyday activities has focused on the experiences expressed through

interviews. There has been less emphasis on the organisation of actual participations and collaborations in activities in real time.

Thus, this chapter will lay out and discuss the practical details of how
such participations and collaborations are shaped and practiced; challenges
and solutions emerging in interactions with people with dementia will be
highlighted. Interaction is also described within the theoretical framework of
emergent pragmatics, where the collaboration and distribution of knowledge and abilities are essential. Among the findings put forward in the chapter are the ways of mobilising resources by participants – including people
with dementia – as well as the type of linguistic and non-linguistic structures
of actions and recurrent interactional patterns the participants in those
activities employ to collaboratively achieve them. The chapter concludes
with a discussion of empirical findings in relation to what and how people
with dementia may contribute to daily activities and what may be expected
of them in terms of their potentialities for being active participants in daily
activities.

In Chapter 7 social psychologist Lars-Christer Hydén shows how collaborative everyday storytelling involving persons with dementia serves as a way to
present and negotiate identity, as storytelling has proved to be one of the most
promising ways to understand meaning-making practices such as identity creation. Of particular importance are the compensatory strategies the participant
uses in order to overcome the challenges presented by the dementia disease.
Although identity often is seen as an individual phenomenon, identities are
shared between persons, for instance spouses. Instead of taking the individual
with dementia as the typical case, it could be assumed that couples in which
one spouse is diagnosed with dementia would present a different picture with
regard to identity and identity change. Presenting, sustaining and negotiating a
shared identity could be seen as part of dynamic, complex and constantly re-
negotiated relationships between the spouses in the couple – made more complicated by the disease.

Telling stories may have many functions but one central function is the presentation and negotiation of identities. People who live together and share a
history, and thus memories, tell stories jointly: stories are thus interactive accom-
plishments and as such they can tell us a great deal about the way we together
create a sense of self. Telling stories is a way for individuals to present and
negotiate their individual identities; when couples or families tell stories together,
it is a way for them to set forth their shared (interdependent) identity. When one
family member develops a dementia disease, this person will face challenges in
taking part in storytelling events and thus in presenting and negotiating stories
through storytelling. Persons with dementia, couples and families develop various strategies in order to be able to continue their storytelling. The strategies
and consequences of shared storytelling that includes persons with dementia
are the focus of this chapter.

In Chapter 8, nursing researcher Ingrid Hellström and social work researcher Annika T. Larsson discuss the significance of relations in order for people with dementia to sustain a sense of agency and self throughout the course of the disease. A general understanding seems to be that people with dementia run the risk of losing their identity and personhood, and that it will lead to a total dependency; *vulnerable* and *dependent* are words commonly used to describe persons with dementia. However, an understanding of everyday life with a dementia disease needs to be anchored on an understanding of relatedness because intimate relationships between the person with dementia and his or her significant others and primary caregivers are instrumental to maintaining a sense of agency and self in dementia. Existing empirical work suggests that 'multi-dimensional and dynamic inter-relationships' between the person with dementia and his or her significant other or carer occur throughout the entire experience of dementia. A number of authors have explored the relational elements of caring in dementia from the perspective of the caregiver (usually it is the spouse who is labelled 'caregiver'). These studies have shed some light on the 'interactive personal experiences' involved, highlighting the fact that most carers (spouses) invest considerable efforts in sustaining the self-esteem and sense of agency of the person with dementia, even if their actual contribution to the relationship diminishes over time. In most caring relationships, the main motivation throughout the entire process is to 'maintain the involvement' of the person with dementia by creating ways in which the person's sense of agency and self can be sustained for as long as possible.

The chapter begins with a theoretical overview of the relational elements in earlier studies on caring in dementia. Based upon empirical research, examples are provided of how people living with dementia can maintain involvement in everyday life at home, even in the later stages of the disease, through relationships and varying, changing and creative forms of interaction with family members and formal caregivers in the form of personal assistance. The chapter concludes with implications for clinical practice and research in the area.

In Chapter 9, occupational therapist Parvin Pooremamli discusses how identity is affected through everyday life at various forms of residential care and also focuses on how the transition to residential care might affect and contribute to a transformation of relations and the trajectory of identities of persons with dementia and their significant others. In later stages of the illness, many people with dementia live at some kind of residential-care facility. The obvious focus of such care facilities is to provide care to the person with dementia, to help them in their daily life with chores it is assumed they no longer are able to do for themselves. However, the manner in which such care is organised has proved important in regard to issues of identity. Studies of speciality units of dementia care in the United States have shown that physiological and emotional outcomes among the residents are quite different between units that employ a biomedical model (and thus treat both the disease and the person with the disease as pathological) and units that employ person-centred care, with emphasis on the abilities retained by the person with dementia. Likewise, dementia care facilities could have a more specific profile, often based on the goal of providing care that corresponds to certain linguistic or cultural practices. Studies of these facilities have shown that mismatch of languages and people not being able to understand each other could result in unmet social needs, leading to social isolation and limited sensory stimulation, and could in fact be one of the reasons why persons with dementia living in mainstream care facilities are prescribed a higher rate of daytime benzodiazepines than persons living in ethno-specific facilities.

This chapter makes use of data from recent empirical research in order to highlight transformations of relations and issues of identity in regard to leaving one's home and moving into a residential-care facility. At the same time, how various forms of residential care can come to affect this transformation is discussed. What activities one is *allowed* to be part of is discussed in relation to issues of doing, being, becoming and belonging and how these issues affect matters of identity.

Finally, in Chapter 10, ethnologist Linda Örulv explores how organisation around self-help and mutual support among persons with dementia helps them deal with challenges in their new life situation, as well as raising their voices as agents in a public debate. By tradition, most information, patient education and emotional support regarding dementia have been offered mainly or solely to the next of kin of persons with dementia because the persons diagnosed with dementia have been assumed to be more or less passive recipients of care. While increasing knowledge and better diagnostic possibilities have rendered early diagnosis possible, meaning that persons with dementia will come to live longer with their diagnosis, and thus with more experience of how to cope and respond to it, there has been less progress in putting their experiences into use in care planning and policy-making. The chapter illuminates and discusses the emergence of self-help groups, mutual support and organization among people with dementia; it focuses on how people with dementia organise and with joint efforts find ways to deal with the challenges of their new life situation as well as raise their voices as agents in public debate. Similar to Chapter 3, the discussion takes its departure in a citizenship perspective, seeing people with dementia as vulnerable to marginalization while at the same time capable of agency within the boundaries of their condition.

An overview of the available research on dementia self-help groups, patient organizations, project groups and networks involving citizens with dementia is presented. In particular, five aspects are dealt with: access to information, mutual support, knowledge development, problem privilege and identity politics. Further, these five aspects are explored through an empirical case of a small self-help group, consisting of persons with dementia. A discursive construction of a shared-meaning perspective and its inherent possibilities for liberation is discussed as the empirical example helps paint a complex picture involving opportunities and limitations of experiential knowledge, issues of double stigmatization and constructs of being interrelated with other people and with the surrounding society. At the centre is the overarching struggle of retaining citizenship in the face of the evolving disease.

References

Cottrell, V. & Schulz, R. (1993). The perspective of the patient with Alzheimer's disease: A neglected dimension of dementia research. *The Gerontologist, 33*, 205–211.

Ferri, C., Prince, M., Brayne, C., Brodaty, H., Fratiglioni, L., Ganguli, M., Hall, K., Hasegawa, K., Hendrie, H., Huang, Y., Jorm, A., Mathers, M., Menezes, M., Rimmer, E. & Scazufca, M. (2005). Global prevalence of dementia: A Delphi consensus study. *The Lancet, 366*, 2112–2117.

Hughes, J. C. (2011). *Alzheimer's and Other Dementias.* Oxford: Oxford University Press.

Schilbach, L., Timmermans, B., Reddy, V., Costall, A., Bente, G., Schlicht, T. & Vogeley, K. (2013). Toward a second-person neuroscience. *Behavioral and Brain Sciences, 36*, 393–462.

WHO (2016). *Dementia.* www.who.int/mediacenter/facts/fs362/en/. Accessed 12 December 2016.

2

TOWARDS A PHENOMENOLOGICAL CONCEPTION OF THE SUBJECTIVITY OF DEMENTIA

Lisa Folkmarson Käll

Conditions of dementia are commonly conceptualised in terms of severe and irreversible loss. In particular Alzheimer's disease, but also other forms of dementia, is associated with a loss of identity, with no longer remembering who one is or recognizing one's surroundings, one's friends and close relatives; with losing one's autonomy, integrity and control of one's actions and existence; with needing help with very basic and intimate needs and thereby also losing one's dignity. Ultimately, dementia is often understood as resulting in a loss of self or of the person while the body lives on as an empty shell. In much recent literature, such a view of dementia is seriously challenged and people with dementia are giving voice to experiences of being selves living with conditions of dementia. Christine Bryden, who has written extensively about her own experience of living with dementia, calls the conception of dementia as leading to a loss of self 'a toxic lie' that makes dementia such a feared condition, often thought to be a fate worse than death (2005, p. 156). This 'toxic lie', however, saturates popular discourse of dementia and provides means – albeit toxic – for conceptualising radically altered self-experience. The view of dementia as resulting in a loss of self or of the person while the body lives on as an empty shell comes to expression in no uncertain terms in a suicide note written by 84-year-old Gillian Bennett, who had lived with and suffered from dementia for three years before taking her own life. She had talked through her decision with her husband and two adult children and they fully supported it. According to Bennett's wishes, after her death, her family published the website deadatnoon.com, containing a statement she wrote before she died.[1]

Explaining her decision to commit suicide, Bennett describes her experience of nearly having lost herself and writes that it is obvious that she is 'heading towards the state that all dementia patients eventually get to', no longer knowing who she is and requiring full-time care of a body that will be physically alive but with no one inside. By committing suicide, she writes, she is giving up nothing that she wants: 'All I lose is an indefinite number of years of being a vegetable in a hospital setting, eating up the country's money but having not the faintest idea of who I am.' In her statement, Bennett expresses clearly a dread of losing control and she writes that she wants to die before she has lost the ability to assess her situation and to take action herself to bring her life to an end. A premonition of a loss of dignity also comes to expression clearly in Gillian Bennett's statement as well as in interviews with her husband and children, who stress that her suicide was a way for her to have a dignified end to her life. It is the condition of dementia, rather than the suicide, that is portrayed in terms of tragedy, something that is also reflected in reactions from readers of the *Vancouver Sun* coverage of Bennett's suicide. Bennett's decision to end her life is met with understanding and even admiration (although she herself in her suicide note denies that it should be an act of courage), far from the discourse of tragedy, flight and the failure of the surroundings that is often articulated in relation to other suicides. The very notion that suicide to avoid the assumed horrors of living with dementia is framed as understandable and rational is testimony to the view of dementia as a condition so horrifying that even death is preferred.[2]

The conception of dementia as leading to a gradual disappearance of the person or the self, while the body as a physical entity lives on, gives rise to a number of interesting and quite urgent questions of what it means to be a person, to lose oneself and to have a body or be embodied. What might it mean to speak of losing one's self? What is this self that is supposedly lost and who is losing this self? This chapter addresses such questions and maps out different conceptualisations of subjectivity or selfhood and of what makes up a human being. First, I briefly present two perspectives on subjectivity or selfhood that in different ways constitute often taken for granted points of departure for predominant understandings of conditions of dementia, such as Alzheimer's disease, namely a dualistic conceptualisation, which draws a distinction between body and mind, and a monistic-materialistic perspective, which views the human being in terms of physical processes. Second, I discuss a phenomenological perspective, which takes its point of departure in the view of human existence as an embodied self that is situated in and as part of a surrounding world and in relation with other embodied beings.

Dualism and monistic materialism

The idea that dementia implies a gradual loss of selfhood and that the body remains as an empty shell rests on a dualistic understanding of the human being in terms of an inner consciousness, mind or soul and an outer body, where it is the inner that is seen to make up a person's identity and subjectivity. We all know this dualistic structuring well and it underlies common conceptions of what it means to be a person. Further, consciousness, and thereby the person, is often conceptualised exclusively in terms of cognition so that the decline and loss of cognitive abilities, as happens in conditions of dementia, are assumed to lead to a loss of subjectivity and identity and a death of the self or a mental death before a death of the body or a physical death.

The dualism between body and mind is perhaps most commonly associated with the French philosopher René Descartes (1596–1650), who famously argues that the body and the mind or the soul make up two completely different substances. The being of the body is extension *(res extensa)*, it has a spatial existence and can be measured and weighed, while the being of the mind or soul is thinking *(res cogitans)* and lacks spatial existence (1982, 26–30, §60–65). The human being consists of both body and mind or soul but that which makes up her person or subjectivity, that which makes her a human person and not simply a mechanical body, is her mind and that she is a thinking being. The person for Descartes is *res cogitans*. Even if body and mind or soul are closely interconnected in human existence, they could potentially, according to Descartes' substance dualism, exist in isolation from each other. For Descartes, the soul, and thus the person, is immortal and therefore cannot be completely annihilated no matter how damaged the body is.

In the Cartesianism that has developed after Descartes and in many ways simplified (and even to some extent distorted) his philosophy, the question of the immortality of the soul or mind is often absent, and it is the dualism between body and mind that is in focus. It is this dualistic conception of the human being that anchors the notion that the mind can be annihilated as a result of dementia while the body lives on as an empty shell. It is this view that Fontana and Smith give expression to when they characterise persons with dementia in terms of 'emptiness behind the facade' (1989, p. 40) and that Bennett puts forth in her contention that throughout the progression of dementia, her body will be physically alive but 'there will be no one inside'.

A dualistic view of human existence is often articulated in terms of a problem of how mind and body interact. The mind-body problem remains unsolvable as long as body and mind are understood as radically different substances, exclusive of one another and functioning according to different laws, that is, a body that is tied to physiology and obeying the laws of nature and a mind that only functions according to free will. Often interaction is framed in terms of causality, as a question of how neurological processes in the brain and nervous system can give rise to conscious states that in turn cannot be completely reduced to such processes. But if the problem of dualism is about how mind and body interact, why make such a strict distinction between mind and body in the first place? The problem seems to be the distinction itself. That the split between mind and body is problematic is obvious in different experiences of one's own body as conscious or of consciousness as altogether bodily. Everyday experiences of one's own lived body are not mainly that of an outer shell for an inner mind, but rather that body and mind are fundamentally a unified whole. This is also something that comes to expression in Bennett's description of her experience of living with dementia and of losing herself; despite her contention that she is losing herself while her body lives on, Bennett nevertheless describes her loss of self as a loss of a unified whole and her 'mindless body' as herself.

In contrast to a dualism between body and mind, a monistic perspective rests on the idea that there is only one type of being. Monistic approaches are often materialistic and understand both body and mind in terms of material processes, either through an understanding of everything as reducible to material processes or by conceptualising body and mind as two aspects of one and the same underlying substance. A monistic materialism thus avoids the problem of how body and mind interact by understanding these in terms of the same substance and as following the same laws of nature. However, even though materialistic perspectives often aim at bridging a dualism between mind and body, they risk giving rise to a new form of dualism, namely that between the brain and the rest of the body. An identity theory of mind or reductive materialism, for instance, claims that the mind is identical with the brain but commonly neglects any discussion of the body other than the brain and makes an implicit distinction between the body and the brain. Mind is understood completely in terms of neurological processes in the brain with the assumption that the mind will deteriorate in cases of deterioration and damage to the brain, as in the case of conditions of dementia. Also, an identity theory can reach the conclusion that a body can live on as an empty shell without a mind if the brain deteriorates because, according to such a theory, the deterioration of the brain is also the deterioration of the mind. Such a view of the mind in terms of neurological processes in the brain has serious implications for understanding conditions of dementia in so far as these involve different forms of damage to and deterioration of brain tissue, which would accordingly entail a corresponding deterioration of the mind.

While materialistic perspectives escape the dualistic problem of interaction between different substances, they give rise to other problems, first and foremost by reducing mental processes to material processes and thereby neglecting the subjective aspects of such processes, what in philosophy of mind is called *qualia*. To neglect the subjective experience of mental processes is to neglect the very meaning of what it is to be conscious; it is the insight that thoughts, feelings and experience cannot be reduced to physical processes that makes dualism and a focus on the irreducibility of the mind persist. Subjective *qualia*, such as the smell and taste of freshly brewed coffee or the feeling of joy, grief, hunger or pain, cannot be caught in objective descriptions and cannot be observed from an outside perspective. The German philosopher Gottfried Wilhelm von Leibniz (1646–1716) describes the irreducibility of *qualia* by asking us to imagine a machine that produces thoughts, feelings and perceptions and that is big enough for us to step inside, the way we can step inside a windmill (2014, §17). If we step inside this machine, writes Leibniz, we will not find the thoughts, emotions or perceptions that it produces; the only thing we will be able to see are different physical constructions that in different ways interact with one another. He argues that in the same way, we will never be able to observe mental states, or *qualia*, when we examine a brain. Regardless of how sophisticated are the tools that we have at our disposal, we will only be able to observe physical processes. The first-person perspective of mental states cannot be reduced to or fully caught by descriptions from a third-person perspective. There are also good reasons as to why consciousness, mind, or soul, and *qualia* are often conceptualized in terms of something inner that exists independently of any outer influence. We all have the experience of being private beings and of having thoughts and feelings that we keep hidden inside us.

Embodied and situated subjectivity

Even though the view of the person with dementia as slowly deteriorating towards a complete loss of herself and subjected to a mental death before physical death dominates cultural and social as well as scientific discourse, it is also, as already mentioned, greatly contested. Much empirical research over the past two or three decades has demonstrated that cognitive and other mental abilities remain throughout the progression of dementia and that conditions of dementia develop without any diminishment of consciousness.[3] Such findings demand different theoretical frameworks and tools for conceptualising personhood and subjectivity than those of dualism and materialism.[4] While a focus on remaining abilities contributes in significant ways to a better understanding of what it might mean to live with conditions of dementia, it might nevertheless risk upholding a dualistic structuring of the human being, with the one, albeit crucial, difference that an inner mind or consciousness is assumed to survive the diminishment of cognitive abilities. Conceptualising the person with dementia in terms of what still remains throughout the progression of cognitive decline involves a risk of reproducing the idea of subjectivity and the person as something inner, separate from the body as an outer shell. In order to avoid such risks and be able to reconceptualise the person with dementia in more comprehensive ways, we must think through more thoroughly what it means to be a self, living as embodied and situated in relation to a surrounding world shared with others.

In addition to the existing rich empirical research on living with dementia, there is also theoretical work from a variety of different perspectives and philosophical frameworks inquiring into subjectivity in relation to dementia and taking embodiment and situatedness into serious consideration. One point of departure for such theoretical inquiry is phenomenology, which offers a framework for approaching issues of embodied situated subjectivity. A particularly useful conceptual tool is the phenomenological notion of the *lived body* (*Leib, corps vécu*), first described and investigated at length by the German phenomenologist Edmund Husserl (1859–1938). The lived body is intended to capture the body as it is subjectively lived and experienced in contrast to the body as an object for the natural and medical sciences (*Körper*) (Husserl, 1989). The notion of the lived body is thus well suited to contest a bio-medical model of dementia accounting only for the deterioration of the brain and the degeneration of cognitive functions. By shifting focus from the brain as the locus of the emergence of personhood to the person as an embodied experiential unity, a phenomenology of the lived body offers a way out of a contemporary hypercognitive culture, marked by a preoccupation with cognition as the defining character of a human being and, as a consequence, dehumanising persons with different forms of cognitive impairment. This preoccupation with cognition as the defining feature of a human being involves a move to pathologise any brain injury in terms of cognitive impairment. In a framework of hypercognition and view of the person in terms of cognition, cognitive impairment is by definition an impairment of the person.

The notion of the lived body bridges the distinction between body and mind without – and in contrast to materialism – reducing one to the other. Instead, the point of departure is that the lived body constitutes a particular type of being and that the distinction between body and mind is secondary and a conceptual abstraction. The notion of the *lived body*, in particular as it has been developed in the writings of the French phenomenologist Maurice Merleau-Ponty (1908–1961), forms one of the starting points, together with Pierre Bourdieu's writings on habitus, for Pia Kontos' influential work on the embodied selfhood of persons with dementia (Kontos 2004, 2005, 2012). Also the notion of *intercorporeality* found in Merleau-Ponty's later writings (1968), which develops the notion of the *lived body* by taking into consideration the constitutive interrelation between bodies, has proved useful for theorising embodied interaction and sociality of persons with dementia (Käll, 2015, 2017; Zeiler, 2014). Both Merleau-Ponty and Simone de Beauvoir (1908–1986) conceptualise the lived body in terms of situation (Merleau-Ponty, 1962; de Beauvoir, 2010) and thereby put focus on social, cultural, historical and material conditions of embodied subjectivity at any given point in time and across temporal duration involving both continuity and change. Here I will discuss two aspects of the lived body that are specifically relevant for approaching subjectivity in relation to conditions of dementia and contesting an understanding of dementia as leading to a complete loss and unbecoming of the self, namely the lived body as a unique singular subjective perspective on the world and the relationality and intersubjectivity of embodied subjectivity.

The lived body, or the embodied subject that Merleau-Ponty also speaks of, constitutes a subjective perspective on the world that is at the same time an object that can be perceived by others. Lived embodiment cannot be made to fit fully in the category of either subject or object and, as Donn Welton points out, when experiencing one's body subjectively, although it seems to belong more to the category of the subject than the object, it can also seem 'to be suspended precariously between them both' (1998, p. 181). As simultaneously both subject and object, the lived body is not in the world as other things are in the world but should instead be understood as being intentionally directed towards and in interrelation with the world of which it also forms part. Husserl famously describes the lived body as the zero-point of orientation (1989, p. 165f) and thereby illustrates how the moving perspective of the lived body constitutes the central point from which the world opens up and receives meaning. The lived body is 'the bearer of the here and the now,' the source in relation to which 'not only what actually appears but to [which] each thing that is supposed to be able to appear' has its orientation (1989, p. 61). The 'here' of which the lived body is the bearer is an absolute 'here' in the sense that it is always 'here' and can never be a 'there'. The lived body is not the zero-point in objective space but the zero-point from which objective space unfolds. In line with this idea, both Merleau-Ponty and de Beauvoir emphasise how lived embodiment is irreducible to an isolated psycho-physical unity and situated in a surrounding world. To be an embodied subject is to be a lived relation with the world through which both one's own bodily subjectivity and the world continuously emerge in relation to one another.

This mutual becoming of embodied subjectivity and its world is perhaps more urgently made manifest when the relation in one way or another is transformed and there is a break in habituated and taken for granted ways of being in and experiencing the world, something that often happens in illness or injury. The onset of a throbbing headache, for instance, can suddenly make ordinary daylight tormenting and enhance bodily tensions and alter comportment and ways of moving in the world. The disorientation associated with conditions of dementia makes the world appear in new, unfamiliar and perhaps frightening ways, which in turn might lead to the lived body losing its habituated ways of being in and relating to the world. It may become more hesitant and insecure, stumbling and staggering, or passive and still. It may no longer trust the world as its point of support or itself as the zero-point of orientation and it may need to develop new perceptual norms and ways of being in the world. According to this view of the embodied self and its relation to the world, a person's surroundings, for instance where she lives or works, form her bodily being, but the surroundings are at the same time also formed by how they are approached by specific people.

A phenomenological perspective on the person as an embodied subject in lived relation with the world dismisses any conceptualisation of the body in terms of a shell, a container or material ground for the mind. Further, in the same way as the lived body cannot be understood as a mere vessel for the mind, the world cannot be reduced to simply a container for the lived body. And, it would be equally misguided to view the mind as a vessel for either body or world. To speak with Merleau-Ponty, 'We have to reject the age-old assumptions that put the body in the world and the seer in the body, or, conversely, the world and the body in the seer as in a box' (1968, p. 138). Such a perspective on subjectivity as essentially embodied and embedded in a world and not reducing the body to an outer shell can thereby contribute to bringing to light and understanding changes that arise in relation to conditions of dementia in terms other than those of mental death before bodily death. Rather than being seen in subtractive terms, such changes may be conceptualised in qualitative terms and as affecting the whole person and her way of being in the world. A view of the lived body as a unique perspective on the world that cannot be caught in objective descriptions takes seriously the presence of a first-person perspective that in the progression of conditions of dementia experiences the changes involved, even when these include disorientation and no longer knowing oneself or recognising one's close friends, relatives or familiar surroundings in the same way as one used to. With the onset of dementia and through the progression of the condition, the lived first-person perspective on the world is not diminished but, rather, altered as relations to the world and others are altered. Through such alterations of the lived first-person perspective there is nevertheless continuity, testified to precisely in the experience of living through the alterations. While this experience involves the experience of loss, as familiar ways of dealing with the world and relating to oneself and others are lost, there is still a first-person perspective of living through that loss.

Dementia and lived embodied subjectivity

The presence of a first-person perspective is brought out nicely in the documentation of the very first case of dementia diagnosed by Alois Alzheimer in 1901 (Maurer & Maurer, 2003). This case was that of the 51-year-old woman Auguste Deter, who displayed unusual behaviour, including confused sense of time and place, incoherent speech and loss of short-term memory. Alzheimer was struck by what appeared to be the degeneration of mental capacities observed in senility but in this case at a much earlier age. He made several clinical interviews with Auguste Deter and after his departure, in 1902, from the asylum in Frankfurt where she resided, he continued contact with the asylum, inquiring about the development of her condition. Upon receiving the news of her death in April 1906, Alzheimer had Deter's medical records and brain sent to him in Munich, where he was then working with psychiatrist Emil Kraepelin. Alzheimer examined Deter's brain using a staining technique to identify so-called amyloid plaques and neurofibrillary tangles, and in November 1906 he presented his findings of the pathology and clinical symptoms of presenile dementia, which Kraepelin later termed Alzheimer's disease.[5] In his file over the case of Auguste Deter, Alzheimer notes 'Instead of "Mrs. Auguste D." she wrote "Mrs."; the rest she had forgotten and had to be told over and over again. As she wrote she said repeatedly, "I have, so to speak, lost myself"' (Maurer & Maurer, 2003, p. 8). While Deter's words of having lost herself mirror the widespread conception of Alzheimer's disease as resulting in a dissolution or loss of selfhood, her words can also be read as testimony that this is not in any way a simple loss. What is striking in her words is not immediately the lack of selfhood, of which she speaks, but, rather, the urgent presence of a self, experiencing the loss of her own self. Deter gives expression to a unique and irreducible subjective first-person perspective on the world and on her own self-experience of losing herself.

Gillian Bennett also writes in her suicide note that she has almost lost herself and gives expression to a first-person perspective experiencing this loss. While Bennett has a quite fixed view of the constitution of the human being and of the effects of conditions of dementia, forming her rational line of argumentation, she does not discuss at any length her actual experience of losing herself and she does not reflect on who this self is who has nearly lost herself. Her statement gives rise to the pressing question of who it is that experiences the disappearance of herself if the person indeed were to disappear as a result of progressive dementia. If the person indeed did disappear and the body was left behind as an empty shell, there would be no one there who, from a first-person perspective, could experience herself as gone. It would in principle be the same as dying or ceasing to exist as a person in the world and thereby no longer having any experiences, positive or negative, of one's condition. The horror associated with conditions of dementia seems not only to be about gradually losing oneself, but also, and perhaps mostly, about the experience of losing oneself, of no longer being oneself or knowing who one is. That fear is to some extent not at all about a mental death before physical death but instead about survival and a continued life in which one experiences oneself in drastically altered form and is perhaps also reduced and dismissed by others as a nonperson or an empty bodily shell. The question of who it is that experiences her own loss of self in dementia, that is, the question of the surviving and irreducible first-person perspective or zero-point of orientation, is an important question to ask, since it draws attention to the person in dementia and highlights that dementia is not something that people simply fall victim to and passively endure but instead something people live with and actively experience.

The lived relation between the embodied self and the surrounding world furthermore also involves a lived relation to other people, that is, other lived bodies or embodied subjects who become who they are in relation to one another. Phenomenology draws attention to the relationality and intersubjectivity of the lived body or embodied self and demonstrates how a singular first-person perspective of one's own embodiment always involves the experience of being intersubjectively accessible precisely as embodied. How the self experiences her own lived body is intimately tied to how she experiences her own body as it is open for the experience of others. Lived embodiment, writes

Merleau-Ponty, reveals with clarity that the order of the subjectively experienced and that of the intersubjectively accessible call for one another and that 'to feel one's body is also to feel its aspect for the other' (1968, p. 137). The way one's body is perceived, understood and assessed by others will undoubtedly have an impact on the way it is subjectively experienced and lived. The lived body is not only the outside manifestation of subjective intentions, but also a site for the inscription of social and cultural norms and values that the self incorporates into who she is and her own embodied self-experience. A culture of conceptualising Alzheimer's disease and other conditions of dementia in terms of loss of self-hood not only, as Athena McLean points out, makes it rather easy for caregivers and others to disregard the agency of persons with dementia 'under the assumption that the actual *person* is gone and that it is the disease that is mean-inglessly acting' (2007, p. 3), but also in harmful ways affects the person living with a condition of dementia. The way in which a person with dementia risks being reduced to the label of a stigmatising disease and thereby be depersonal-ised and invalidated through the often unintentionally harmful behaviour of healthy others is brought to light by what Tom Kitwood terms 'malignant social psychology' (1997, p. 14). Such malignant social psychology can be seen when the primary focus for others' interaction with a person with dementia is the disease rather than the person, something that risks leading to the erasure of personal characteristics and silencing transformation of self-expression into symptoms of cognitive decline. While we must never fail to recognise and respect that there may be a significant difference between the way a person lives her life and the way someone else might see her way of living, we must at the same time also recognise how subjective self-experience is never isolated but instead formed in a social and cultural context. By putting focus on the relationality and intersubjectivity of lived embodiment, a phenomenological framework demonstrates relationality as essential to human existence and therefore as something that must be taken into serious consideration when giv-ing an account of how conditions of dementia affect subjectivity and self-experience. People with dementia must, as Julian Hughes et al. put it, 'be understood in terms of relationships, not because this is all that is left to them, but because this is characteristic of all of our lives' (2006, p. 5).

Questions of loss

In addition, the meaning of loss in the view of dementia as resulting in a loss of self can be fruitfully rethought from a phenomenological perspective that draws attention to subjectivity as relational and in continuous becoming. In discus-sions about the supposed loss of self in the progression of conditions of demen-tia there is an underlying assumption of what might be called a subtractive conception of loss, according to which loss entails a subtraction of a part from something whole, leaving that whole incomplete, reduced or diminished. This form of subtractive view of loss is clearly at the root of Fontana and Smith's claim that as Alzheimer's disease develops 'there is less and less' of the self left 'until where once there was a unique individual there is but emptiness' (1989, p. 45). Also Gillian Bennett gives expression to a subtractive conception of loss when she writes that within a limited amount of time of living with progressive dementia, she will no longer be here and that her mind will eventually be totally gone. The loss of self is conceptualised as a subtraction from an original whole that after subtraction is left diminished and incomplete. Such a subtractive view of loss not only presupposes an original whole from which something is subtracted, but also assumes that this whole is static, denying a view of the self as continuously changing and becoming a self.

The experience of losing oneself while still remaining a self who is experiencing one's own loss of self requires other ways of conceptualising loss. Here, a phenomenology of embodied subjectivity can help us make sense of loss not primarily in quantifiable terms of subtraction but instead in qualitative terms of alteration. By emphasising the relationality of embodied subjectivity and conceptualising its being in terms of becoming, a phenomenological perspective rejects any idea of the identity of subjectivity as a stable whole and thereby also calls into question the possibility of understanding loss of self as a subtraction of a part from such an original stable whole. If the self is not an atomistic entity with clearly defined boundaries, a loss of self cannot be thought of in terms of a simple subtraction from an original whole. Instead, loss may be thought of as resulting in a qualitative restructuring of the self so that the self after loss is qualitatively different from what it was but not necessarily diminished or incomplete. In an understanding of selfhood as relational and self-relational, continuously becoming itself in a process without completion, loss in fact appears as an integral part of the becoming of the self and thus as an element of its constitution. In each moment of becoming who one is, there is an alteration of selfhood that entails an ongoing loss of who one was even though the past of what one was at the same time remains as a trace in the movement of becoming. Such an understanding of self-loss as constitutive of the being of the self is brought forth by the Swiss philosopher Rudolf Bernet, who writes that 'one's own selfhood is ultimately nothing other than the capacity of the subject for loss of the self' (1996, p. 170). The self is here understood as a structure of loss through its relationality and alteration. The loss of self is thus constitutive of selfhood so that the self would not be a self at all without this element of self-loss in each moment of its becoming. In such a view, selfhood cannot be understood in terms of an atomistic and isolated whole and loss of self cannot be reduced to a matter of simple subtraction. Instead, the being of the self is conceptualised in terms of becoming and loss of self is a qualitative feature of self-becoming.

A conceptualisation of subjectivity in terms of loss and alteration could provide a productive way of challenging too simple a conceptualisation of loss and of better understanding experiences of loss of self as a result of conditions of dementia. Clearly, there are losses involved in experiencing the progression of dementia and in receiving a dementia diagnosis. The recorded words of Auguste Deter speak of such experience, as do the final words of Gillian Bennett and the words of others describing their experiences of living with dementia. However, as testimonies of loss of self also demonstrate, such losses can never be understood in any simple way of subtraction. The challenge when approaching a popular conception of dementia as leading to a loss of self is perhaps not to struggle over whether the self loses her self but to think through different forms of loss of self in relation to one another. Alterations that happen in conditions of dementia are *both* a matter of severe loss, of no longer being who one is, *and* a matter of remaining who one is, living through loss and finding ways of reorientation and rehabituation. An understanding of the loss of self as an integral element of selfhood might serve to de-stigmatise the deep forgetfulness that accompanies the onset of dementia and to establish a sense of continuity between that which passes unmarked as 'normal' subjectivity and that which is marked and pathologised as the subjectivity of dementia. A phenomenological approach to selfhood, drawing attention to the self as embodied and situated, in continuous becoming in relation to itself, others and its surrounding world, not only has implications for understanding the person with dementia as living through the condition and being a self experiencing her own loss of self, but also opens for care practices that start from the self in terms of becoming and as fundamentally relational rather than as an isolated and atomistic subject.

Conclusion

How we decide to conceptualise subjectivity, body and mind in relation to dementia has both ethical and political implications. Gillian Bennett was quite clear that she saw her suicide as an ethically defensible alternative, perhaps the only ethically defensible alternative, in light of her situation. The ground for her view, motivating her decision, was a crass dualistic view of the human being and an equally crass understanding of the outcome of progressive dementia. The case of Bennett's suicide puts focus on the ethical implications of the well-established understanding of dementia as a slow deterioration and disappearance of the person that leaves the body behind as an empty shell. If the person is gone and only an empty shell remains, what reason could we have to keep that empty shell alive? What could even in such circumstances legitimate keeping the empty shell alive? And who would then be able to exercise rights, get good care and be met with respect and dignity?

In contrast to established dualistic and materialistic perspectives, a phenomenological understanding of embodied subjectivity implies that the person is not reduced to a cognitive inner core and thereby that the whole person, not only her cognitive capacities, can be met. Loss of cognitive function does not, therefore, in a phenomenological framework, automatically lead to a disappearance of the person since the person is understood in terms of lived embodiment, situated in a world and interrelated with others. While dementia, without a doubt, involves thoroughgoing changes of a person's situation and how one's own bodily subjectivity is lived and experienced, these changes do not imply that the person is no longer situated in relation to her surroundings or lives and experiences her own embodiment and situation. Indeed, regardless of how it plays out, life involves changes of situations, relations and experiences. A phenomenological perspective that sees bodily subjectivity as an active and ongoing relation to the surrounding world can also better make sense of and conceptualise the disorientation that often follows from dementia. Disorientation thereby does not necessarily appear as a sign of an unambiguous loss of identity and anchoring in the world but can instead point to a continued but drastically altered relation to the world. Such a perspective also opens the possibility of different forms of reorientation and new ways of being in the world and living with dementia.

Notes

1   Gillian Bennett committed suicide on 18 August 2014. Her posthumously published webpage, www.deadatnoon.com, includes links to media coverage on Bennett's decision to end her life, and her suicide note was published also, by the daily newspaper *Vancouver Sun*. A compilation of the articles published in the *Vancouver Sun* is available here: www.vancouversun.com/news/topic.html?t=topic&q=gillian+bennett.

2   Dementia also often leads to anticipatory grief, that is, grief over someone even before that person has died, which can contribute to increasing stigmatisation and to a strengthening of the idea that dementia is equal to a mental death before physical death. See Rando, 1986.

3   See Hedman, 2014; Hughes et al., 2006; Hughes, 2011; Hydén et al., 2014; Kitwood, 1997, 2007; Kontos, 2004, 2005; Sabat, 2001a, 2001b; Sabat & Harré, 1992; Örulv, 2008. For an overview of conceptualisations of subjectivity in relation to Alzheimer's disease, see Herskovits, 1995.

4   Indeed, both dualism and materialism appear quite insufficient to account for embodied subjectivity and the experience of embodied existence, whether with or without a condition of dementia. A conscious lived body that everyone who is embodied knows to be a factual reality turns out to be a theoretical impossibility if mind and body are defined as separate irreconcilable substances or if one is reduced to the other.

5   The diagnostic term Alzheimer's disease was until the 1970s used only to refer to *pre*senile dementia but was at that time grouped together with late-life or senile

dementia as the latter was medicalised. The medicalisation of senility has, as Elizabeth Herskovits writes, been 'accepted and widely popularized through the proliferation of Alzheimer's disease' (1995, p. 149). Nowadays, Alzheimer's disease refers predominantly to senile dementia whereas cases of presenile dementia of the Alzheimer type are often termed early-onset Alzheimer's disease.

References

Beauvoir, S. de. (2010). *The Second Sex*. Translated by Constance Borde and Sheila Malovany-Chevallier. New York: Alfred A. Knopf.

Bennett, G. 2014). Goodbye and Good Luck! www.deadatnoon.com. Accessed 12 December 2016.

Bernet, R. (1996). The other in myself. In Simon Critchley & Peter Dews (Eds.), *Deconstructive Subjectivities*. Albany, NY: SUNY Press.

Bryden, C. (2005). *Dancing with Dementia*. London: Jessica Kingsley Publishers.

Descartes, R. (1982). *Principles of Philosophy*. Translated and with an introduction by Valentine Rodger Miller and Reece P. Miller. Dordrecht: Kluwer.

Fontana, A. & Smith, R. (1989). The 'unbecoming' of self and the normalization of competence. *Sociological Perspectives, 32*, 35–46.

Hedman, R. (2014). *Striving to be able and included: Expressions of sense of self in people with Alzheimer's disease*. Stockholm: Karolinska Institutet.

Herskovits, E. (1995). Struggling over subjectivity: Debates about the 'self' and Alzheimer's disease. *Medical Anthropology Quarterly, 9*, 146–164.

Hughes, J. (2011). *Thinking Through Dementia*. Oxford & New York: Oxford University Press.

Hughes, J., Louw, S. & Sabat, S. (2006). Seeing whole. In Julian Hughes, Stephen Louw & Steven Sabat (Eds.), *Dementia: Mind, Meaning and the Person*. Oxford & New York: Oxford University Press.

Husserl, E. (1989). *Ideas Pertaining to a Pure Phenomenology and to a Phenomenological Philosophy*. Second Book: Studies in the Phenomenology of Constitution. Translated by Richard Rojcewicz and André Schuwer. Collected Works, Volume III. Dordrecht: Kluwer.

Hydén, L. C., Lindemann, H. & Brockmeier, J. (Eds). (2014). *Beyond Loss: Dementia, Identity, Personhood*. Oxford & New York: Oxford University Press.

Kitwood, T. (1997). *Dementia Reconsidered: The Person Comes First*. New York: Open University Press.

Kitwood, T. (2007). In Clive Baldwin & Andrea Capstick (Eds.), *Tom Kitwood on Dementia: A Reader and Critical Commentary*. New York: Open University Press.

Kontos, P. (2004). Ethnographic reflections on selfhood, embodiment and Alzheimer's disease. *Ageing and Society, 24*, 829–849.

Kontos, P. (2005). Embodied selfhood in Alzheimer's disease: Rethinking person-centred care. *Dementia 4*, 553–570.

Kontos, P. (2012). Alzheimer expressions or expressions despite Alzheimer's? Philosophical reflections on selfhood and embodiment. *Occasion: Interdisciplinary Studies in the Humanities 4*, 1–12. http://hdl.handle.net/1807/72006. Accessed 11 February 2017.

Käll, L. F. (2015). Intercorporeal relations and ethical perception: Portrayals of Alzheimer's disease in *En Sång för Martin* and *Away from Her*. In Aagje Swinnen & Mark Schweda (Eds.), *Popularizing Dementia: Public Expressions and Representations of Forgetfulness*. Bielefeld: Transkript Verlag.

Käll, L. F. (2017). Intercorporeal expression and the subjectivity of dementia. In Luna Dolezal & Danielle Petherbridge (Eds.), *Body/Self/Other: A Phenomenology of Social Encounters*. Albany: SUNY Press.

Leibniz, G. W. (2014). *Leibniz's Monadology: A New Translation and Guide*. Translated by Lloyd Strickland. Edinburgh: Edinburgh University Press.

Maurer, K. & Maurer, U. (2003). *Alzheimer: The Life of a Physician and the Career of a Disease*. New York: Columbia University Press.

McLean, A. (2007). *The Person in Dementia: A Study of Nursing Home Care in the US*. Toronto: University of Toronto Press.

Merleau-Ponty, M. (1962). *Phenomenology of Perception*. London & New York: Routledge.

Merleau-Ponty, M. (1968). *The Visible and the Invisible*. Evanston, IL: Northwestern University Press.

Örulv, L. (2008). *Fragile Identities, Patched-up Worlds: Dementia and Meaning-Making in Social Interaction*. Linköping: Linköping University.

Rando, T. (1986). *Loss and Anticipatory Grief*. Lanham, MD: Lexington Books.

Sabat, S. (2001a). Surviving manifestations of selfhood in Alzheimer's disease: A case study. *Dementia, 1,* 25–36.

Sabat, S. (2001b). *The Experience of Alzheimer's Disease: Life Through a Tangled Veil*. Oxford & Malden: Blackwell.

Sabat, S. & Harré, R. (1992). The construction and deconstruction of self in Alzheimer's disease. *Ageing and Society, 12,* 443–461.

Vancouver Sun. www.vancouversun.com/news/topic.html?t=topic&q=gillian+bennett. Accessed 12 December 2016.

Welton, D. (1998) Affectivity, eros and the body. In Donn Welton (Ed.), *Body and Flesh. A Philosophical Reader*. Malden & Oxford: Blackwell Publishers.

Zeiler, K. (2014). A philosophical defense of the idea that we can hold each other in personhood: Intercorporeal personhood in dementia care. *Medicine, Health Care and Philosophy, 17,* 131–141.

3

DEMENTIA IN THE AGE OF MIGRATION: CROSS-CULTURAL PERSPECTIVES

Eleonor Antelius

Introduction

Back in the 1980s, a cross-cultural collaboration of several scholars from around the world initiated project AGE, to shed light on how different sociocultural settings come to shape the experience and meaning of (successful) aging (see e.g. Fry et al., 1997). This has since been further developed, both in practice – where both ethnogerontology and ethnogeriatrics are now common in many care education's curricula – as well as in gerontological research, where preeminent researcher Sandra Torres has published substantially on the issue at hand (see e.g. Torres, 2002, 2004, 2015; Torres & Hammarström, 2009; Torres & Lawrence, 2012). What is argued is that the way in which people regard ethnicity has implications not only for how gerontological research is designed but also for how policies for old age are formulated and how gerontological practice is shaped. As one of gerontology's guiding principles, however, 'successful aging' is still very much a debated concept, not the least because it has failed not only to acknowledge that old age is in fact a social construction but also that it is rooted in a Western tradition, in which non-Western understandings are seldom taken into consideration (Torres, 2001, 2004; Torres & Hammarström, 2009, p. 25). For instance, in many Western countries one often talks about 'the third age' – that is, when one is no longer working full time but is in such good health that one can manage on one's own – suggesting a new time of self-fulfilment, with an increased freedom to consume both experiences and products. Aging well in such a society thus often means to be able to stay independent and have the means and resources to fulfil oneself. In other societies, this is not how one ages well. Take, for instance, an example from ethnographic studies in rural Jamaica (Bourne, 2009), where it has been shown that old age is associated with an increased status, resulting in increased social connections, which in turn transforms into receiving more assistance from other people. Thus, with increased age comes the incentive that you should not have to do things for yourself anymore and should have someone do it for you, leaving you sitting still a lot more and gaining weight and thus also being unable to achieve current fashion ideals. Hence, the lived experience of growing, and getting old, differs in historical and cultural contexts, just as studies have also shown how differences in perceptions and experiences of growing old affect individuals' help-seeking behaviour and their inclination to use or not use formal care services.

The need to understand the wider process of aging as well as more 'distinct' diseases such as the dementias as socially and culturally constructed is thus imperative when one also brings into discussion the fact that we live in 'the age of migration'. In 1993, Stephen Castles and Mark Miller published the innovative book *The Age of Migration: International Population Movements in the Modern World*, discussing international migration flows and the impact such flows could have on ethnic relations in different societies. Although some demographers at the time questioned if the twentieth century could indeed be called 'the age of migration' (see e.g. Torres & Lawrence, 2012), the influx in migratory movements in the early twenty-first century, with more than 60 million people estimated to be on the run from conflicts, war or terror, certainly has strengthened Castles and Miller's thesis on migration as a global 'trend'. More and more societies are affected by migration and transnationalism and more and more people from different social and cultural backgrounds will be born in one country but live out their elderly days and end of their lives in another. This means that in most nations around the world today, there will most likely exist many varying definitions of what dementia 'is': how it is perceived and experienced as well as how it will affect what people expect when growing old.

It has been 30 years since Sharon Kaufman wrote her book *The Ageless Self: Sources of Meaning in Late Life*, but still it illustrates why it is imperative to remember what old age – and successful aging – could mean:

> In order to improve the quality of life experience for those in their later years, we must understand what it means to be old.... Only by knowing how the elderly view themselves, their lives, and the nature of old age can we hope to fashion a meaningful present and future for them and those who follow. (Kaufman, 1986, p. 4)

As Kaufman and many other scholars before and after her have argued, aging and old age must be understood from 'within', from the voices and perspectives of those who actually are old and live with diseases such as the dementias. Hence, in order to discuss dementia, and old age, in relation to migratory contexts, this chapter will discuss cross-cultural perceptions of the dementias as well as highlight certain features from a specific case-in-point of ethnocultural contextualisation of dementia care through interviews and discussions with Middle Eastern immigrants.

Varied responses to dementia

International studies show that as people tend to live longer, in both industrialised and developing countries, more people will live into old age and as such have a higher risk of developing an age-related dementia disease. As mentioned in the introduction in this book, WHO estimates that the number of people living with dementia worldwide is currently 47.5 million, a number predicted to double by 2030 and almost triple by 2050 (World Health Organization & Alzheimer's Disease International, 2016). This demographic trend is often discussed as being a challenge from an economic perspective, putting pressure on governments, policy makers and other stakeholders to address the impact of dementia as an increasing threat to global health (ibid).

Alongside being an issue of economics, dementia has historically also been portrayed as an issue of 'social suffering'. Although this book highlights and puts forward a much more contemporary, agentival approach in which the person with dementia is understood in relation to the people surrounding her rather than one isolated individual with a 'dysfunctional' brain, one question still often raised regarding chronic diseases, such as dementia diseases, is whether there exists variation by ethnic groups. Although there is strong evidence that both genetics and environmental factors most likely play significant roles in determining risk, for instance, of Alzheimer's disease (Larsson & Imai, 1996), the prevalence of dementia diseases has proved to be quite similar in different parts of the world. Dementia seems to affect all groups equally, with no known links to either geographical location or specific ethnic groups (Cayton, Graham & Warner, 2006). However, how people *respond* to such diseases has proved to be quite diverse; responses are often culturally distinctive and linked to how people understand and experience diseases such as the dementias (Antelius & Plejert, 2016; Valle, 1998, p. xix).

Thus, besides the economic and political impact, the expected increase in the number of people developing dementia diseases will also pose a challenge in terms of coping with complex and varied responses to dementia that could be grounded in culture. Perceptions of dementia diseases can thus be regarded as social representations; that is, perceptions that are shared with other people belonging to the same group, society or culture rather than being individual entities. Social representations thus make it possible to create meaning in illnesses; why do they exist, how do they occur, how do we cure them (if possible) and how do we respond to them. In the Western world, which is strongly influenced by a biomedical worldview, there is a strong tendency to perceive dementia as being caused by neurofibrillary tangles and plaques (i.e. the pathological causes of a deteriorating brain) with symptoms often associated with loss of cognitive functions such as lost memories and the ability to remember, but also to be able to think, and act, rationally. However, social representations are perceptions that are shared with other people and thus necessarily will be quite varied depending on historical and cultural context. This means that the biomedical definition of plaques and tangles, of reduced cognitive functioning and declining rationality, are not universally applicable.

Cross-cultural perceptions of dementia

Several scholars have shown that although it may be possible to arrive at a common biomedical definition of dementia (or at least of Alzheimer's disease), the symptoms and experiences associated with the disease are plentiful, and alternative interpretations and experiences of dementia can be profound (Traphagan, 2009). For instance, Lawrence Cohen (1995, 1998) was one of the first to ethnographically study functional decline in later life. In the mid-1990s, he started researching issues related to elderly persons in India and was able to show that the symptoms usually gathered under the generic term dementia were not perceived or described at all as they were in his home country, the United States. The elderly people he met and studied in India who experienced deteriorating memory, had difficulties orienting in time and space and had developed problems in communicating were not considered to suffer from any (brain) disease. Instead, their 'problems' were believed to be caused by bad family relationships (Cohen, 1995, 1998). As such, Cohen was one of the first to show how culturally constructed notions of madness, old age and senility were intertwined with a moral subtext of what constitutes good (or bad) behaviour, rather than just being a disease inside one's skull.

Cohen's research has been followed by a few other scholars, such as John Traphagan (2002, 2005, 2009), who has studied the meanings associated with loss of brain function and how this is manifested within the cultural context of contemporary Japan. Traphagan was able to show how *boke* (a Japanese term that resists any easy translation but could be thought of as somewhat like senility) is best understood as a moral category, because *boke* (senility) is something one should be able to control by means of mental and physical efforts. In Japanese, the human nature is often described with two words, *kokoro* (the inner heart) and *karada* (the outer body); the outward appearance is part of human behaviour, and the mind should control the body. To not be able to control one's body is thus in some ways one's own fault, as one has not kept fit. Hence, *boke* represents a state where one has 'given up' any attempt to keep one's mental health (Anbäcken, Minemoto & Fujii, 2015). As such, *boke* (or senility, or dementia) is not so much a biomedical definition of a disease as it is a moral concept indicating you have let yourself go.

Other studies show that dementia is perhaps not understood as a disease at all but rather as 'normal aging'. For instance, Olson (1999) has shown that among Hmong Americans (Americans of Hmong descent from Southeast Asia), 'dementia' is not considered a serious condition; rather it is perceived as a natural part of the life cycle, and for such conditions, one need not seek treatment. Similarly, Gerdner, Xiong and Cha (2006) have shown that Hmong immigrants who experience confusion and memory loss in old age are treated by shamans using traditional approaches (such as the use of herbal tea and medicinals), often leading to better ways of coping with the symptoms (p. 30).

Scholars such as Neil Henderson (2002, 2015; Henderson & Henderson, 2002; Henderson & Traphagan, 2005) and Kristen Jacklin (Jacklin, Pace & Warry, 2015; Jacklin, Waker & Shawande, 2013; Jacklin & Warry, 2012) have shown how hard it is to 'translate' similar symptoms from one cultural context to another. Although not being perceived as 'normal aging', confusion and forget-fulness might not always be interpreted as abnormal either. Instead, Henderson and colleagues, who have studied Native American tribes in the United States, as well as Jacklin and colleagues, who have studied First Nation members in Canada, have been able to show how such symptoms could in fact be under-stood as a 'supernormal state'; a state where the experiences and behaviours of the person with dementia are perceived as spiritual encounters with the afterlife and thus more as positive experiences than pathological behaviours.

The multidimensionality of dementia

Examples such as these are among a growing number of studies signifying that dementia is always experienced within a convergence of personal and social stories; of values, norms and traditions as well as individual and shared experi-ences. Thus, whatever diseases such as the dementias are, they are multidimen-sional, and dementia thus also needs to be understood as a lived experience rather than simply a biological fact. In other words, dementia needs to be de-medicalized in order to facilitate an extended analysis of dementia models in which social and cultural factors such as recognition of symptoms, help-seeking strategies, caregiving and coping could become more apparent (Antelius & Traphagan, 2015; Henderson, 2002). As stated above, in biomedical terms dementia is defined as irrevocable cognitive decline caused by microscopic changes of plaques and neurofibrillary tangles in the brain. By tradition this is also how most of the research concerning persons with dementia has been framed: as a progressive brain disease that occurs within a person's skull. Hence, research regarding persons with dementia has often focused upon individuals and their (declining) cognitive abilities. This of course is beneficial in terms of understanding dementia as a progressive brain disease but not quite as helpful if we would like to try to understand how people with dementia live and cope with their illness (Hydén, 2014). To put it in the words of scholar Kay Toombs (2001a, 2001b): the definition of a disease seems to explain very little and cap-tures little, *if anything*, of the actual experience of living with an illness.

As a consequence, it has been argued that it is of immense importance that persons with dementia diseases be understood not only as isolated – sick – indi-viduals with nonfunctioning brains but also as persons who belong to a social context, interacting with other people. A shift in research concerning the socio-cultural research regarding dementia has indeed occurred; for a number of years now, there has been a rapidly growing field of dementia studies that goes beyond the individual's loss and instead understands dementia not only as a biomedical disease but also as a subjective experience that incorporates both personhood and identity in complex terms of transformation and change. Significant in this approach is that the disease cannot be solely understood as 'trapped' inside the brain of the person with dementia. Instead, it understands the transformations and changes brought about by the disease as collaborative (Hydén, 2014; Hydén, Lindemann & Brockmeier, 2014). Hence, the importance of understanding that persons with dementia diseases are not isolated – sick – individuals with nonfunctioning brains, but persons who belong to a social context, in which interactions with other people have been strongly stressed (Hydén & Örulv, 2009; Kitwood, 1997; Lyman, 1989; O'Connor et al., 2007; Örulv, 2008). Thus, we have seen how studies of dementia have turned away from the definitions of a disease process, towards a more in-depth understanding of the fact that a person with dementia is just that, a *person*, who lives in close relations to others and engages in interactions with other people.

Normal ways of being ill

Still, however, when social context has been taken into account, it has often been regarded as the immediate, personal surroundings of the person living with dementia, giving the illusion of dementia as 'occurring in a vacuum' (O'Connor et al., 2007). One could indeed speak of a tendency to ignore the importance of larger sociocultural contexts, such as values, norms and beliefs; this is highly problematic because we have seen above that different ethnocultural groups could ascribe different meanings to the illness (see also Dilworth-Anderson & Gibson, 2002; Leibing & Cohen, 2006 for further discussion regarding these issues). These ascribed differentials have been shown to affect not only how a person living with Alzheimer's disease or another dementia is perceived and what status is afforded to the ill person (Antelius & Traphagan, 2015; Dilworth-Anderson, Williams & Gibson, 2002; O'Connor et al., 2007) but also if one is inclined to use formal services or not (Connell et al., 2009; Flaskerud, 2009; Gray et al., 2009; Hinton, Franz & Friend, 2004).

Hence, in order to more fully understand the complex social contexts that individuals with dementia are part of, we need to pay more attention to the fact that the way people understand and explain health and illness is always culturally (and socially) shaped. To borrow a classical idea from anthropologist Arthur Kleinman (1988): we need to understand that there are always *normal ways of being ill* and that such normal ways will most often result in very different health-maintenance and help-seeking behaviour. Understanding this point thus has significant implications, not the least from a clinical perspective, as clearly, dementia is not simply a (biomedically defined) pathology of the brain but also a disease that is highly culturally demarcated and socially shaped.

When considering how dementia is expressed and experienced, it has thus proved necessary to give some thought to how people in a given context think about the nature of a human being. In what ways are concepts of self and person defined in the context in question? How do we perceive the construction – and the deconstruction – of the self (as dementia has often been perceived as being such 'deconstruction')? These are questions that are crucial to ask, and to understand; as the perception of the self has been shown to be closely connected to how the care provided is organized (Antelius & Traphagan, 2015).

Aging multicultural populations

Most nations today have experienced rapid population growth and have been affected by large-scale migration (immigration as well as emigration), meaning that most nations become more and more multicultural (Castles & Miller, 2003). Hence, many nations are experiencing an increasing number of immigrants – with culturally and linguistically diverse backgrounds – growing old in their 'new' country of residence (see e.g. Emami & Ekman, 1998). Put in relation to what has been discussed above, the experience of – and response to – diseases such as the dementias may vary distinctively depending on worldview, norms, traditions and values.

'Normal aging', as well as 'successful aging', needs to be understood not just from its historical context but also its sociocultural context. The 'third age' discussed above, when elders are supposed to experience a new time of self-fulfilment and an extended freedom, is by no means the established norm for all elders. For instance, in interviews conducted with Persian immigrants living in Sweden, it turned out that most often adult children decided to cease caregiving at home and seek formal residential care for their elderly parents with dementia; the elderly themselves had very little to do with this decision. However, this is very much at odds with Swedish policies concerning care assessment, according to which it is the person with dementia who should be the one at least consenting to the formal decision (Kiwi, *forthcoming*). In the discussions with the children who had made these decisions (sometimes even by 'tricking' their parents that they were indeed moving back home to Iran), it turned out that the children – of course – did not do this out of spite or because they believed their parents incapable of making these decisions on their own but rather because it was their duty to do so. In their upbringing, they had been taught to take care of their elderly, implying not just actual physical caring but also taking responsibility for and making decisions concerning their wellbeing (Kiwi, *forthcoming*).

Ethnocultural contextualisation of dementia care

Generally speaking, one could say that larger studies of ethnoculturally profiled dementia care facilities are (extremely) scarce. The few studies that are more substantial (that go beyond a single individual paper or two) have until now been undertaken mainly in Sweden (by Ekman 1993; Ekman et al., 1993, 1994) or in Australia (see Runci et al., 2005a, 2005b, 2012). However, also in the Swedish and Australian studies, the ethnocultural aspect has remained in the background, leaving the linguistic aspect of profiled care on centre stage, where results show that people who live with dementia diseases functioned on a level of manifest competence that seemed far below their level of latent competence when interaction was based upon the person with dementia's second language rather than their native tongue. However, people living with dementia who resided in a profiled care home where staff spoke the native tongue of the residents seemed better off, participated more in conversations and general interaction and were prescribed fewer antianxiety medications. In regard to what most of the chapters in this book discuss, that cognitive resources are not just individual but rather created in relation to other, supporting, partners, this is not all that surprising; a common language most likely supports such successful interaction. However, studies have yet to show if an ethnocultural profile of the residential home where one resides with people of the 'same' origin and with similar cultural backgrounds does as well. And still, in response to the development of dementia care policies, in the last few years several so-called ethnically profiled dementia care facilities have emerged in Sweden. These are residential-care facilities that state that they are different from ordinary municipal care facilities in that they offer something more – or rather something *else* – by being targeted towards specific ethnocultural groups. For instance, *Anahita* (the fictive name of one such residential-care facility) states the following:

> Anahita is a Persian facility for those of you who long for home in your elderly days. At Anahita we do not just speak Persian. When you arrive at Anahita we want to create a sense of being 'home in Iran'. We have decorated with furniture, carpets, aromas, paintings, and other things reminiscent of the homeland. There are smaller sitting groups for drinking tea as well as possibilities to smoke the water pipe. We have all the classic party (parlor) games, Persian TV, Persian radio, Persian music. Here at Anahita we show respect and consideration for the different view on gender existing in the Persian culture. For elderly persons with Muslim background it can be important to be cared for by someone of the same sex. Family is important. When you move to Anahita we are foremost a complement to your own family. We will not take over. Your family will still be able to have responsibility.

It is quite clear from this short description of *Anahita* that *home* is depicted as something other than Sweden: 'when you long for home ... being home in Iran'. It seems as if 'home' is where one has one's cultural roots, where

everything seems to be different from the Swedish version of the same phe-
nomena: there are Persian TV, Persian parlour games, Persian music, Persian
decorations, Persian smells, etc. There is a Persian way to understand family
relations and the role of the care staff; gender issues will be dealt with differently
than in contemporary Sweden. And all of this will be incorporated into the care
of the elderly with dementia diseases at *Anahita*. However, what is not explained
in the above description of *Anahita* is how one perceives diseases such as the
dementias. How are they understood, explained and experienced? And, how
could this perception come to affect the notion of 'being home in Iran'?

The following part of this chapter uses examples that stem from research project
Ethnocultural Diversity and Dementia Diseases which is part of research programme
Dementia, Agency, Personhood & Everyday Life (RJ M10:0187-1) to illustrate cross-
cultural perspectives of dementia and utilisation of dementia care (see
e.g. Antelius & Kiwi, 2015; Antelius & Plejert, 2016; Antelius & Traphagan, 2015;
Kiwi, Hydén & Antelius, *(in review)* Strandroos & Antelius, 2016) and to further discuss and problematise cross-cultural perspectives of dementia and dementia care.

Special recognition should be given to PhD candidate Mahin Kiwi who has collected
and used much of the data in her own analysis in her forthcoming dissertation
Dementia or "loss of memory" among elderly Iranian immigrants living in Sweden.

Varied understandings of dementia

In interviews with care staff, participants, residents and relatives at day centres,
residential-care homes and in-home help services targeted towards Middle Eastern immigrants living in Sweden, we found that the perception of what dementia is varied considerably:

Example 1.

Arif: Relatives of those coming here have become <u>a little</u> more aware, they
             have more knowledge about the disease, but in the beginning they
             knew nothing of dementia. So it is … a little bit of bad knowledge about
             dementia diseases among our people from the Middle East, really bad
             knowledge. … In general, they connect this disease with old age, if
             you're old, of course you forget.

I: Ok, so it becomes natural when one—

A: You know, it's natural but it's not at all natural. We have young people
             with dementia, under the age of 65 here, that's not natural. It's a disease
             really, but for them it's connected to, well, being old they say.

Example 2.

Interviewer: I hear that you say dementia. Is that a common term in Iran or Kurdistan?

Ayda: No, what we call dementia here [in Sweden] is called Alzheimer's in Iran.

I: Do people know what Alzheimer's is?

A: No, they don't.

I: What do they call it?

A: In Kurdish they call it khérfé [crazy/lunatic].

I: Does that mean that a person's ability to understand is constantly decreasing?

A: Exactly. Sometimes one says that s/he has lost his/her mind and intelligence ... One feels sad when hearing someone describe a demented person as being without intelligence.

Example 3.

Shila: What is characteristic for people with dementia diseases is in elderly in Iran called senility or in the worst case lunatic or something like that. What is called dementia in Sweden is called khereft [fool] or mentally ill in Iran.

None of the interviewees used any Persian, Kurdish or Azerbaijani terms when talking about the disease, even if the interview was conducted in the respective language. They all used either the Swedish term 'demens' (dementia) or said 'memory loss' rather than 'dementia'. This indicates that dementia – or any other term describing the same condition – is not common in conversations in Persian (or Azerbaijani or Kurdish). Similarly, participant observations showed how care staff usually did not perceive the residents as having a disease; rather they explained the residents' actions as 'daydreams', questioning if the residents are perhaps just burdensome and troublesome because they have always been like that. Dementia, it turned out, was seldom perceived or described as a disease at all. Instead, a more open questioning of the term was common:

Example 4.

Shervin, 52:   I honestly do not know if either staff or relatives have any idea what dementia is.

Example 5.

Ayeh, 57:   Frankly, none of us know what dementia is.

Varied understandings – and experiences – of dementia care

Several studies have shown that the way that people ascribe meaning to a disease (such as the dementias) could have a bearing on health-maintenance and health-seeking behaviour as well as the inclination to use formal services (see e.g. Botsford, Clarke & Gibb, 2011; Conell & Gibson, 1997; Daker-White et al., 2002; Dilworth-Anderson & Gibson, 2002; Dilworth-Anderson, Williams & Gibson, 2002) meaning that the perceived perspectives of dementia described above could influence how, and whether, people with such perceptions seek formal care services. However, in our studies we found very little evidence for this causal logic. Instead, it seemed as if it was not always the ascribed meaning of the disease that had a bearing on health-seeking behaviour and the inclination to use formal services but rather the care service form itself.

Example 6.

Shiva: We are all Iranians and we still live with the Iranian culture, which complicates things around us. According to Iranian culture, we have not yet figured this formal care out.

Interviewer: I have often heard that Iranians are ashamed to place their parents in residential care, is that right, do you think?

S: Yes, there is some truth in that, but it is not the relatives that are ashamed of their decisions but the parents who end up in the residential home. The parents are the ones having trouble accepting that their children have turned them over to the hands of social welfare authorities and not manage to care for them themselves. The very concept of a residential home is burdensome and difficult to understand for those elderly who have children, whom they have given all their support so that one day they can take care of them. ... I know many who don't want to live here as they perceive it to be weird and unnatural.

Example 7.

Farbia: We are often ashamed to tell our friends and family that mother is living in an institution. I understand relatives that are ashamed of this because their parents built their future and now it's their time to reap what they have sowed.

As previous studies have shown (e.g. Chang et al., 2011; Kwon & Tae, 2012), filial piety is often perceived and experienced as much stronger among minority groups. For instance, Abdollahpour et al. (2012) state that strong emotional bonds between families have demarcated Iranian society, where taking care of one's parents has been one of the major duties of families. However, Abdollahpour and colleagues also describe how this has started to change, due to factors such as urbanisation, smaller families, longer life expectancies and large-scale migration (p. 545). The influx of other cultural norms and traditions seems important to acknowledge in order to not just reproduce 'old' ideas about filial piety. However, there is also one other aspect that further complicates this notion of filial piety as the 'sole cause' of hesitation regarding formal care services, one which has not been dealt with to any extent in previous literature, namely believed causes of dementia:

Example 8.

Afsoon: During the time I have lived in Sweden I have never heard of anyone in the family [back in Iran] who has gotten Alzheimer's. As everyone live together all the time, one does not get dementia.

Example 9.

Amira: It's not easy now, for our family. My mum and dad after 60 moved to Sweden, completely foreign country. It's not easy for them, and I understand one becomes depressed and demented after some years because they can't accept, they feel like prison, they can't go any-where, don't feel ... uhm, they don't know the language, don't dare to go out, they are just home, home, home. And we work so we can't be there all the time. After a few years most will become demented.

Interviewer: Like faster [than native Swedes]?

A: Aa, much faster. Because you leave your country, all you have fought for and then, suddenly you have to leave and go to another country and know nothing. We who are young can learn the language, and work and all that, but those who come after 50–60 years of age, it's not easy for them ... after a short while you get this disease.

I: So the new social circumstances make you ill quicker?

A: Aa, because in our home countries we just go out and there is a lot of people in the roads and you talk and time flies and you just go out and say hello and socialize with neighbours ... help out, have coffee together. ... [W]e have more social. ... [B]ut when they come here they don't see any people and the winter is dark and cold and ... several days perhaps, they don't meet anyone and they don't go out ... so one just sits and thinks and thinks and thinks.

Example 10.

Hadya: It's hard bringing an old into a new culture, new country, new language ... really hard. Myself I came when I was 25 and I still feel ... don't blend in in society, uhm, so, how's it when they are 60–70–80? But sometimes you have to bring your [parents], they have nothing left, you can't leave them alone.

Interviewer: So, what's it like when they come here? Can you give an example?

H: Yes, the old you mean?

I:	Yes.
Hadya:	I knew some who … uhm, they couldn't do anything, they became depressed, they were trapped … uhm, it's like you say, you take a fish out of the ocean … that's how it is for older people. There they had a life of their own, they had youth, friends, colleagues, they went to the cafés, they talked. But then they come here, they only know their children who works all day … they have nowhere to go.…You know, we use such proverb, one takes a fish, this fish out of water and place it somewhere else [where it does not belong] so even if they did not have diseases they might get them here because they are lonely, loneliness.

These longer examples are provided in order to illustrate the perception of dementia as possibly being caused by loneliness and isolation (or even by the migration itself) due to the fact that one has left one's 'natural habitat' (as explained with the proverb about the fish). However, this also indicates that dementia needs to be understood as something one can prevent: if you are not alone you will not attract such diseases. Hence, formal services are perhaps not only perceived as shameful in the sense that one has abandoned old traditions and customs according to which the family is obliged by filial piety to take care of their elderly, but are also seen as causing (or enhancing) the disease because the person with dementia is thought to be more isolated and lonely in formal care than in family care. The disruption of cultural continuity, it seems, also is perceived as a probable cause of illness (and dementias), and isolation stemming from migrating in old age enhances the likelihood of getting a dementia disease. Similarly, formal residential care seems able to make a person even more ill:

Example 11.

Fariba:	If you say that *nn* is forgetful and that it is deepening and deepening one gets to hear, oh no, Mother didn't used to be forgetful. She became like this while in residential care.

Example 12.

Shervin:	Relatives will not accept the truth. They say: last year Mother was able to cook for herself, but since she came here, she can't even walk on her own.

Discussion

Earlier research has shown how different ethnocultural settings shape the experience and meaning of aging as well as dementia diseases and how different perceptions and ascribed meanings of a disease can affect health-maintenance and health-seeking behaviour. And yet, most studies regarding dementia place the person with dementia within a so-called 'personal vacuum', that is, in disregard of the fact that all people, also those with dementia diseases, are part of larger sociocultural contexts, where values, norms and beliefs will come to influence how one perceives, experiences – and responds to – the illness (Antelius & Plejert, 2016).

Hence this chapter has explored the understanding of dementia as a culturally and socially shaped illness in order to illuminate perceptions of as well as experiences of and responses to both dementia and dementia care. The case-in-point has been to do so in regard to ongoing studies of persons with Middle Eastern background partaking in ethnoculturally profiled dementia care in Sweden. With that said, I believe that it is crucial to discuss the fact that in many countries around the world, it is quite common to inform and educate care staff with the help of so-called resource kits (i.e. written guides concerning cultural profiles of different ethnocultural groups). These kits are to be used by staff within aging-care services in order to improve quality of care and best practice in regard to the aging multicultural population. Alzheimer Australia was the first to publish such kits, and they have since been spread worldwide and translated into several languages. These kits all stem from the original Australian one (URL 1) and are translated and (supposedly) adapted to the particular country's circumstances after 'feedback from representatives from each population' (URL 2). However, when looking at, for instance, the Danish version of the kit, one soon notices that it is almost identical to the Australian one. In regard to, for instance, the 'cultural profile of the Arabic-speaking community', which outlines perceptions of dementia and attitudes towards residential care, it is hard to spot anything particularly 'Danish' in the cultural profile of the Arabic-speaking community in Denmark.

The constant flux of culture

Given that the empirical examples above showed that the perception of dementias and the described meaning of have diseases have little (or nothing) to do with decisions regarding formal care, it could be helpful to introduce the concept of acculturation, that is, the theory surrounding changes that come about when people come in contact with other cultures (as introduced by Redfield, Linton & Herskovits in 1936) in order to better illuminate issues regarding ethnoculturally profiled care. *The acculturation continuum* (Valle, 1998) is a means of trying to explain one's degree of ethnic identification and was developed to try to help practitioners to respond appropriately to cultural variations encountered when working with ethnoculturally diverse groups (ibid). The continuum goes from a traditional position, characterized by the preservation of cultural origins, to bicultural positions marked by persons moving with relative ease between both cultures, to the end of the continuum, where one more or less identifies with the new society's cultural norms (Valle, 1998; Yeo & Gallagher-Thompson, 1996). Previous studies have shown how degrees of acculturation could be linked to changes in health behaviours as well as changes in knowledge and beliefs (see e.g. Landrine & Klonoff, 2004).

One could perhaps state that some of the persons in the examples above show tendencies of rejecting their 'original' culture and adopting a Swedish culture of defining dementia as a disease. As Arif above put it: we did not know anything about it at home, but now we know that dementia is *not* something natural, it *is* a disease and people from the Middle East need to understand such (which Arif and several of the other interviewees suggested they did not). However, interviewees also described some people with Middle Eastern background (mainly those with Arab background) as being more traditional in regard to retaining cultural origins than *other* Middle Eastern immigrants. For instance, Mitra, an assistant nurse, stated:

> I believe, through my own experience and by talking to others who also feels the same way, that Arabic-speaking people are more willing to take care of their elderly at home by themselves and it is part of the culture. Yet, such is indeed the case for us Iranians as well but I think that its, in Sweden perhaps we Iranians have *adapted* us.

What Mitra thus points to is that it seems hard to believe that immigrants with Middle Eastern background now living in Sweden (or any other country they might have migrated to for that matter) will automatically have the same attitude towards residential, formal care as immigrants with Middle Eastern background in Australia did (where the above discussed resource kit originated), simply based upon the fact that they have migrated from the same area and might (or might not) have had similar perceptions and experiences of dementia (and dementia care) in their home country. As Mitra states, and the acculturation theory suggests, people adapt and change in relation to surrounding society. In regard to the resource kit, which was almost identical in the Australian and Danish versions, it is as if the whole 'Arabic-speaking community' *also* existed in a vacuum, with no regard to the fact that *cultural ideas, norms and traditions change over time and in correlation to surrounding society*.

It might have seemed excessive to use all those empirical examples above, but the examples clearly illustrate that to understand more about immigrants with dementia it is crucial to understand how people perceive, experience and respond to dementia care *within* that new country. An insight recently discussed in a study exploring response processes among Pakistani immigrants living in Norway (Næss & Moen, 2015) illuminates the idea that dementia care – in a migratory context – must be understood in relation to the health-care culture and its system in the 'new' society. Stagnant assumptions based upon some general notion of cultural perceptions of the dementias on a group level will not help at all.

This chapter has thus discussed cross-cultural perceptions of dementia and dementia care and highlighted the importance of never underestimating the impact cultural norms and traditions might have in regard to social interaction, care and care-seeking behaviours. Neither the individual person with dementia nor larger ethnocultural groups can be placed within a vacuum that seemingly does not change or correlate with surrounding society.

Learning outcomes and practical implications

In regard to the empirical examples presented from the research programme *Ethnocultural Contextualization and Dementia Care* and the more general international theoretical discussions on understanding dementia in the age of migration as a socially and culturally constructed concept, some learning outcomes and practical implications can be derived:

1 Perceptions of dementia seem to have little to do with utilisation of formal care services – this is in stark contrast to what many studies from the past have shown.

2 Health-seeking behaviour and utilisation of formal care services seem to be more tied to norms of filial piety, and acculturation also is important: understanding migratory contexts seems more key than understanding preconceived perceptions of the disease itself.

3 However, we must also recognize the fact that believed *causes* of dementia could in fact impact people's utilisation (or nonutilisation) of formal care services.

Thus, in regard to cross-cultural perspectives on dementia, it is crucial to understand that in a time considered to be 'the age of migration', more and more people will move between countries and countries will become more and more multicultural. Thus, to handle a growing number of individuals developing dementia diseases in these countries, individuals and ethnocultural groups can no longer be placed in a vacuum. For all people to be able to age successfully (whatever that may mean to different individuals), we *must* take into consideration people's values, norms and traditions when we think about and design tomorrow's dementia care. And we must remember that values, norms and traditions are in constant flux; perhaps inert, but never static. Hence, the main practical implication for tomorrow's dementia care seems to be to be able to incorporate these two positions, to culturally adapt dementia care at the same time as to not let it stagnate.

References

Abdollahpour, I., Noroozian, M., Nedjat, S. & Majdzadeh, R. (2012). Caregiver burden and its determinants among family members of patients with dementia in Iran. *International Journal of Preventive Medicine, 3,* 544–551.

Anbäcken, E.-M., Minemoto, K. & Fujii, M. (2015). Expressions of identity and self in daily life at a group home for older persons with dementia in Japan. *Care Management Journals, 16,* 64–78.

Antelius, E. & Kiwi, M. (2015). Frankly, none of us know what dementia is: Dementia caregiving among Iranian immigrants living in Sweden. *Care Management Journals, 16,* 79–94.

Antelius, E. & Plejert, C. (2016). Ethnoculturally profiled care: Dementia caregiving among Middle Eastern immigrants living in Sweden. *Anthropology & Ageing, 37,* 9–26.

Antelius, E. & Traphagan, J. (2015). Ethnocultural contextualization of dementia care: Cross-cultural perceptions on the notion of self. *Care Management Journals, 16,* 62–63.

Botsford, J., Clarke, C. & Gibb, C. (2011). Research and dementia, caring and ethnicity: A review of the literature. *Journal of Research in Nursing 16*(5), 437–449.

Bourne, P. (2009). Good health status of older and oldest elderly in Jamaica: Are there differences between rural and urban areas? *Open Geriatric Medicine Journal, 2,* 18–27.

Castles, S. & Miller, M. (2003). *The age of migration. International population movements in the modern world.* [3rd edition]. Hampshire: Palgrave McMillan.

Cayton, H., Graham, N. & Warner, J. (2006). *Alzheimer's and Other Dementias.* London: Class Health.

Chang, Y., Schneider, J. & Sessanna, L. (2011). Decisional conflict among Chinese family caregivers regarding nursing home placement of older adults with dementia. *Journal of Aging Studies, 25,* 436–444.

Cohen, L. (1995). Toward an anthropology of senility: Anger, weakness and Alzheimer's in Banaras, India. *Medical Anthropology Quarterly, 9,* 314–334.

Cohen, L. (1998). *No Aging in India: Alzheimer's, the Bad Family, and Other Modern Things.* Los Angeles: University of California Press.

Connell, C. & Gibson, G. (1997). Racial, ethnic, and cultural differences in dementia caregiving: Review and analysis. *The Gerontologist, 37*(3), 355–364.

Connell, C., Roberts, S., McLaughlin, S. & Akinleye, D. (2009). Racial differences in knowledge and beliefs about Alzheimer disease. *Alzheimer Disease and Associated Disorders, 23,* 110–116.

Daker-White, G., Beattie, A., Gilliard, J. & Means, R. (2002). Minority ethnic groups in dementia care: A review of service needs, service provision and models of good practice. *Ageing and Mental Health, 6*(2), 101–108.

Dilworth-Anderson, P. & Gibson, B. (2002). The cultural influence of values, norms, meanings, and perceptions in understanding dementia in ethnic minorities. *Alzheimer Disease and Associated Disorders, 16,* 56–63.

Dilworth-Anderson, P., Williams, I. & Gibson, B. (2002). Issues of race, ethnicity, and culture in caregiving research: A 20-year review (1980–2000). *The Gerontologist, 42,* 237–272.

Ekman, S.-L. (1993). *Monolingual and bilingual communication between patients with dementia diseases and their caregivers.* PhD dissertation, Umeå University Medical Dissertation, 0346-6612.

Ekman, S.-L., Robins Wahlin, T.-B., Norberg, A. & Winblad, B. (1993). Relationship between bilingual demented immigrants and bilingual/monolingual caregivers. *International Journal of Ageing and Human Development, 37,* 37–54.

Ekman, S.-L., Robins Wahlin, T.-B., Viitanen, M., Norberg, A. & Winblad, B. (1994). Preconditions for communication in the care of bilingual demented persons. *International Psychogeriatrics, 6,* 105–120.

Emami, A. & Ekman, S.-L. (1998). Living in a foreign country in old age: Elderly Iranian immigrants' experiences of their social situation in Sweden. *Health Care in Later Life, 3,* 183–199.

Flaskerud, J. (2009). Dementia, ethnicity, and culture. *Issues in Mental Health Nursing, 30,* 522–523.

Fry, C., Dickerson-Putman, J., Draper, P., Ilkes, C., Keith, J., Glascock, A. P. & Harpending, H. C. (1997). Culture and the meaning of a good old age. In J. Sokolovsky (Ed.), *The Cultural Context of Aging: Worldwide Perspectives* (pp. 99–123). Westport, CT: Bergin & Garvey.

Gerdner, L., Xiong, S. & Cha, D. (2006). Chronic confusion and memory impairment in Hmong elders: Honouring differing cultural beliefs in America. *Journal of Gerontological Nursing, 32,* 23–31.

Gray, H., Jimenez, D., Cucciare, M., Tong, H.Q. & Gallagher-Thompson, D. (2009). The cultural influence of values, norms, meanings, and perceptions in understanding dementia in ethnic minorities. *American Journal of Geriatric Psychiatry, 17,* 925–933.

Henderson, N. (2015). Cultural construction of dementia progression, behavioral aberrations, and situational ethnicity: An orthogonal approach. *Care Management Journals, 16*(2), 95–105.

Henderson, N. (2002). The experience and interpretation of dementia: Cross-cultural perspectives. *Journal of Cross-Cultural Gerontology, 17,* 195–196.

Henderson, N. & Carson Henderson, L. (2002). Cultural construction of a disease: A 'supernormal' construct of dementia in an American Indian tribe. *Journal of Cross-Cultural Gerontology, 17,* 197–212.

Henderson, N. & Traphagan, J. (2005). Cultural factors in dementia: Perspectives from the anthropology of aging. *Alzheimer Disease & Associated Disorders, 19,* 272–274.

Hinton, L., Franz, C. & Friend, J. (2004). Pathways to dementia diagnosis: Evidence for cross-ethnic differences. *Alzheimer Disease and Associated Disorders, 18,* 134–144.

Hydén, L. C. (2014). Cutting Brussels sprouts: Collaboration involving persons with dementia. *Journal of Aging Studies, 29,* 115–123.

Hydén, L. C., Lindeman, H. & Brockmeier. J. (2014). *Beyond Loss: Dementia, Identity, Personhood.* New York: Oxford University Press.

Hydén, L. C. & Örulv, L. (2009). Narrative and identity in Alzheimer's disease: A case study. *Journal of Aging Studies, 23,* 205–214.

Jacklin, K. & Warry, W. (2012). Forgetting and forgotten: Dementia in aboriginal seniors. *Anthropology & Aging Quarterly, 33,* 13.

Jacklin, K., Pace, J. & Warry, W. (2015). Informal dementia caregiving among indigenous communities in Ontario, Canada. *Care Management Journals, 16,* 106–120.

Jacklin, K., Walker, J. & Shawande, M. (2013). The emergence of dementia as a health concern among First Nations populations in Alberta, Canada. *Canadian Journal of Public Health, 104*, e39–e44.

Kaufman, S. R. (1986). *The Ageless Self: Sources of Meaning in Late Life.* Madison: University of Wisconsin Press.

Kitwood, T. (1997). *Dementia Reconsidered: The Person Comes First.* Philadelphia: Open University Press.

Kiwi, M. (*forthcoming*). *Dementia or "loss of memory" among elderly Iranian immigrants living in Sweden.* Linköping: LiU Press. [Doctoral dissertation].

Kiwi, M., Hydén, LC. & Antelius, E. (*in review*). Deciding upon transition to residential care for persons living with dementia: why do Iranian family caregivers living in Sweden cease caregiving at home? *Journal of Cross-Cultural Gerontology.*

Kleinman, A. (1988). *The Illness Narratives.* New York: Basic Books.

Larsson, E. & Imai, Y. (1996). An overview of dementia and ethnicity with special emphasis on the epidemiology of dementia. In Yeo & Gallagher-Thompson (Eds.), *Ethnicity and the Dementias* (pp. 9–20). Washington, DC: Taylor & Francis.

Leibing, A. & Cohen, L. (Eds.) (2006). *Thinking about Dementia: Culture, Loss, and the Anthropology of Senility.* New Jersey: Rutgers University Press.

Lyman, K. (1989). Bringing the social back in: A critique of the biomedicalization of dementia. *The Gerontologist 29*, 597–605.

Næss, A. & Moen, B. (2015). Dementia and migration: Pakistani immigrants in the Norwegian welfare state. *Ageing & Society, 35*(8), 1713–738.

O'Connor, D., Phinney, A., Smith, A., Small, J., Purves, B., Perry, J., Drance, E., Donelly, M., Chaudhury, H. & Beattie, L. (2007). Personhood in dementia care. Developing a research agenda for broadening the vision. *Dementia, 6*, 121–142.

Olson, M. C. (1999). The heart still beats, but the brain doesn't answer: Perception and experience of old-age dementia in the Milwaukee Hmong community. *Theoretical Medicine & Bioethics, 20*, 85–95.

Örulv, L. (2008). *Fragile Identities, Patched-up Worlds. Dementia and Meaning-making in Social Interaction.* Linköping: LiU-Tryck. PhD dissertation, Linköping Studies in Arts and Science No. 428/Linköping Dissertations on Health and Society No. 12.

Österholm, J. H., Tagizadeh Larsson, A. & Olaison, A. (2015). Handling the dilemmas of self-determination and dementia: A study of case managers' discursive strategies in assessment meetings. *Journal of Gerontological Social Work, 58*, 613–636.

Runci, S., Eppingstall, B. & O'Connor, D. (2012). A comparison of verbal communication and psychiatric medication use by Greek and Italian residents with dementia in Australian ethno-specific and mainstream aged care facilities. *Alzheimer Disease and Associated Disorders, 24*, 733–741.

Runci, S., O'Connor, D. & Redman, J. (2005a). Language needs and service provision for older persons from culturally and linguistically diverse backgrounds in southeast Melbourne residential care facilities. *Australasian Journal on Ageing, 24*, 157–161.

Runci, S., Redman, J. & O'Connor, D. (2005b). Language use of older Italian-background persons with dementia in mainstream and ethno-specific residential care. *International Psychogeriatrics, 17*, 699–708.

Strandroos, L. & Antelius, E. (2016). Interaction and common ground in dementia: Communication across linguistic and cultural diversity in a residential dementia care setting. *Health: An Interdisciplinary Journal for the Social Study of Health, Illness and Medicine.* Online First: November 28, as doi:10.1177/1363459316677626.

Toombs, K. (2001a). Introduction: Phenomenology and medicine. In K. Toombs (Ed.), *Handbook of Phenomenology and Medicine* (pp. 1–26). Dordrecht: Kluwer Academic Publishers.

Toombs, K. (2001b). Reflections on bodily change: The lived experience of disability. In K. Toombs (Ed.), *Handbook of Phenomenology and Medicine* (pp. 247–261). Dordrecht: Kluwer Academic Publishers.

Torres, S. (2001). *Understandings of 'successful ageing': Cultural and migratory perspectives.* PhD thesis, Department of Sociology, Uppsala University, Sweden.

Torres, S. (2002). Relational values and ideas regarding 'successful aging'. *Journal of Comparative Family Studies, 33,* 417–431.

Torres, S. (2004). Making sense of the construct of successful ageing: The migrant experience. In S.O. Dattland & S. Biggs (Eds.), *Ageing and Diversity: Multiple Pathways and Cultural Migrations* (pp. 125–139). Bristol: Policy Press.

Torres, S. (2015). Expanding the gerontological imagination on ethnicity: Conceptual and theoretical perspectives. *Ageing & Society, 35,* 935–960.

Torres, S. & Hammarström, G. (2009). Successful aging as an oxymoron: Older people – With and without home-help care – Talks about what aging well means to them. *International Journal of Ageing and Later Life, 4,* 23–54.

Torres, S. & Lawrence, S. (2012). An introduction to 'the age of migration' and its consequences for the field of gerontological social work. *European Journal of Social Work, 15,* 1–7.

Traphagan, J. (2002). Senility as disintegrated person in Japan. *Journal of Cross-Cultural Gerontology, 17,* 253–267.

Traphagan, J. (2005). Interpreting senility: Cross-cultural perspectives. *Care Management Journals, 6,* 145–150.

Traphagan, J. (2009). Brain failure, late life, and culture in Japan. In J. Sokolovsky (Ed.), *The Cultural Context of Aging* (pp. 568–575). Westport: Praeger Publishers.

URL 1: Alzheimer Australia. *Perceptions of dementia in ethnic communities.* www.fightdementia.org.au/files/20101201-Nat-CALD-Perceptions-of-dementia-in-ethnic-communities-Oct08.pdf, accessed 12 December 2016.

URL 2: National Videnscenter for Demens [Danish Dementia Research Center]. *Opfattelse av demens blandt personer med anden kulturel og sproglig baggrund.* [Perceptions of dementia among persons from culturally and linguistically diverse background]. www.videnscenterfordemens.dk/media/1069316/informations%20pjece_hjemmeside.pdf, accessed 12 December 2016.

Valle, R. (1998). *Caregiving Across Cultures: Working with Dementing Illness and Ethnically Diverse Populations.* Washington DC: Taylor & Francis.

World Health Organization and Alzheimer's Disease International (2012). *Dementia: A public health priority.* http://apps.who.int/iris/bitstream/10665/75263/1/9789241564458_eng.pdf?ua=1, accessed 12 December 2016.

4

CITIZENSHIP-IN-AND-AS-PRACTICE: A FRAMEWORK FOR IMPROVING LIFE WITH DEMENTIA

Ann-Charlotte Nedlund and Ruth Bartlett

Introduction

Utilising a citizenship perspective in order to study and problematise situations for people living with dementia has received increasing attention during the last decade. A significant aspect of this perspective is to recognise persons living with dementia as active agents with the right to be self-determining and to exert power over their own lives. For some people with dementia, this means speaking up and speaking out, as Jim Mann (2015), a high-profile international campaigner for Alzheimer Society, Canada, explains:

> … [M]ore and more of us are challenging boundaries and finding our voice. We are 'claiming full citizenship' – speaking up and speaking out, and assuming our place at the table as capable and active participants.

Whilst we recognise that not every person with dementia is able or willing to operate at this level, such practices are important to explore because they are creating possibilities for participation in politics and policy processes that were not there before. In particular, they shed light on how policies are, or at least could be, influenced by the voices of people with dementia.

In this chapter we therefore examine the idea of citizenship *in* and *as* practice as a framework for improving life with dementia. The discussion is organised further into five sections. The first section outlines our reasons for focusing upon citizenship in and as practice, rather than human rights, because this has also received increasing attention during the last decade. The second section introduces the key features of citizenship in and as practice; these are rights, access, belonging and agency. The third section discusses how citizenship in and as practice can be utilised to improve life for people with dementia. The fourth section gives a brief overview of the emerging discourse of citizenship within dementia studies. The fifth and final section considers some of the challenges and tensions of problematising matters within a citizenship framework.

Why citizenship-in-and-as-practice rather than human rights?

As well as citizenship, the discourse of human rights is moving up the agenda in dementia studies. The rights of people living with dementia to live a good life and to be treated equally and fairly are discussed at the highest level of political discourse. For example, the first United Nations-appointed independent expert on human rights and freedoms for older people, Rosa Kornfeld Matte, emphasised in spring 2015 at a World Health Organization (WHO) ministerial meeting the value of paying attention to the human rights of people with dementia (Kornfeld Matte, 2015). At this meeting, she emphasised how the dignity and fundamental human rights of people with dementia should be respected and upheld throughout the dementia journey, and that individuals should have the opportunity to participate in life whenever possible. Rosa Kornfeld Matte (2015) explained that:

> Participation means that people with dementia are entitled to be active, free and in a meaningful manner, participate in, contribute to, and enjoy civil, political, economic, social and cultural lives. People with dementia should remain integrated and included in society and participate actively in the formulation and implementation of policies that directly affect their well-being.

Moreover, she emphasised how people with dementia are likely to need support to exercise and claim their rights, but that their right to autonomy and independence must also be recognised and respected. Similarly, non-governmental organisations in the United Kingdom are outlining the benefits of taking a rights-based approach to improving the lives of people with dementia, and in particular, the opportunities such an approach brings for 'elevating' the collective voice of people with dementia to bring about change (Mental Health Foundation, 2015, p. 22).

So why focus on citizenship rather than human rights? What is the difference between these two equally compelling ideas and approaches? Such questions are important to raise, as the discourses of citizenship and human rights need to be disentangled, for the assets of the former to be seen. According to citizenship scholars, it is not possible to have human rights without first having citizenship. As Shachar (2014) points out: 'our basic right to have rights remains deeply fragile and insecure so long as we can be deprived of membership in an organized political community'. Similarly, Isin and Turner (2007) consider a 'viable state as an important guarantee for rights .... [H]uman rights that cannot be enforced by an authority are a mere abstraction.' Thus, their view is that 'citizenship should be regarded as a foundation for human rights not as a competitor' (Isin & Turner, 2007). It is a view we share; hence, the primary focus on citizenship.

Understanding citizenship and citizenship practice

Why is citizenship of importance in the context of people living with dementia?

It is common for needs to be pathologised when a person has dementia, especially if that person resides in a care home or is in hospital. People with dementia are typically described as having 'symptoms' (rather than rights) and care needs (rather than agency). Take, for example, the reporting of a study recently conducted in Australia on the benefits of Skype conversations for people with dementia. The researchers found that the visual and auditory stimulation of the Skype conversations helped to 'capture the person's attention and reduce agitation' (Van der Ploeg et al., 2016). Although the researchers clearly recognise the value of people with dementia staying connected to family members, a person's right to a family life was not commented upon, and neither was the integral role the person with dementia was playing in that life. In our view, there needs to be a more balanced commentary on life with dementia and how this relates to being and acting as a citizen and enabling citizenship practice as in the example above.

So, in order to analyse dementia and people living with dementia from a citizenship perspective it is essential to understand how the relationship among citizens, and between the state (as well as its institutions and caregiving organisations) and its citizens, is interrelated to practice. Empirical research could assess and reveal actual findings but here we will suggest a framework for understanding these interrelated characters and critically reflecting on how citizenship can be enabled formally and in everyday situations.

The key definitional features of citizenship

In problematising citizenship, we will suggest a framework that is based to a large extent on Wiener's work on citizenship practice in the European union context (1997, 1998, 2013). This approach sheds light on the relational as well as on social constructive aspects of citizenship. In order to get there, we will first present the key definitional features of citizenship that give a constructive base to start an analysis, that is, what Wiener (1997, 1998) explains as the constitutive parts of citizenship and the three core elements of citizenship that are related to citizenship practice. Throughout the text we will present examples for how this framework can be adapted to explore citizenship and its practice in the context of people living with dementia.

To start, citizenship is a relational concept; it encompasses a relationship between the citizens and the community (sometimes referred to as a political entity) and also the relationship between the individual citizens. These are the constitutive parts of citizenship (Wiener, 1998). Accordingly, citizenship can be understood as an agreement between the political community and the citizens and is thus related to ideas and principles of democracy. What they all have in common, however, is to define people as political agents. Normatively, citizenship is related to two different political ideas: the liberal with influences from the Roman model, which emphasises the rights and obligations of the citizens; and the communitarian and civic republican with influences from the Greek model, in which citizenship is the process of governing and being governed and thus the focus is on political participation, self-government and the interests of the wider community (Lister, 2007). Accordingly, there are different normative traditions and ideas, one that focuses on the status as a citizen in a political community and the other that focuses on participation and both of which can be tracked in the notion of citizenship practice.

Also, citizenship is inevitably based on the notion of inclusion and exclusion, in which some groups of people will be inside the community and others outside it, either formally or informally. The relationship between the community and its citizens is constantly under negotiation and therefore under change. On this basis, we can distinguish citizenship as relational as well as continuously defined and re-defined based on social norms and values that construct and ascribe the conditions for citizenship and its practice. As Wiener (1998) argues, every analysis of citizenship has to encompass these three parts: the state (and its institutions), the citizens and the relation between these.

Further, Wiener outlines three core elements that are related to citizenship, which will then help us to understand, explore and enable citizenship practice. These elements are rights, access and belonging.

Rights (to what?)

The first dimension, *rights*, constitutes the formal dimension and can be regarded as individuals' legal connections to society. To that we would add that in order to elaborate on the element of rights, one has to ask 'rights to what?'.

The rights dimension has commonly been associated with Marshall's classical division of citizenship rights into civil, political and social rights (Marshall, 1991/1950), which, he argues, is the basis for citizenship in the Western welfare states. Commonly it is reflected that the third form, the social rights, can encompass many forms of entitlements (cf. Dwyer, 2010). The social rights differ since they also are not as regulated in detail in the constitution as the civil and political rights. Social rights are visible in the constitution more in terms of what the state is responsible for than in terms of rights that the citizens actually legally can claim.

Expansion to rights of anti-discrimination and recognition (Joppke, 2007) in the form of minority rights (also Kymlicka, 1995) targets immigrants and their descendants as well as people with disabilities (c.f. Barnes & Mercer, 2003) and dementia (c.f. Kelly & Innes, 2013; Boyle, 2014). Other types of rights also have been acknowledged, for example economic, cultural and reproductive rights (c.f. Lister, 2009), occupational rights (Townsend & Wilcock, 2004), academic rights (Hakosalo, 2011), language rights (Kymlicka & Patten, 2003), digital rights in terms of online accessibility (c.f. Hafford-Letchfield et al., 2010) and sexual and intimacy rights (Richardson, 1998). What these other types of rights illustrate, and what we think is important to have in mind when understanding citizenship, is that the dimension of rights does not have to follow the division identified by Marshall but can also be expanded to include other types of rights. By doing so, *rights to what* opens up several forms of problematisations when studying citizenship for people with dementia.

Furthermore, political rights require some form of democratic conditions. Democracy is about how power should be distributed and sometimes removed from citizens in terms of 'being ruled' and also 'to rule'. There should be reciprocity in the power relationship between the people who govern and those who are governed, where citizens should have equal access to participation, influence and self-determination. This agreement is what citizenship is about. How this manifests depends on the conditions that actually exist but also on normative ideas about good governance and the good citizen. The basic principle in a democracy is that citizens must in different ways be involved and participate in the political issues that operate in the community. This can be done by voting in elections and accountability in the form of protests (representative democracy), by active membership in associations and direct involvement (participatory) and through deliberations and discussions in which different actors can participate and together arrive at some form of consensus (deliberative democracy). The focus on what political rights are differs somewhat. The two latter highlight the citizen's active participation in politics to a greater extent than simply choosing representatives at elections every four (or some other interval) years. From this follows an idea that citizens should be closer to the decisions made at different levels in society. In other words, different normative ideals, related to different democracy theories about how a society should be organized, highlight different dimensions as desirable in the relationship between government and citizens and between the citizens. Political rights need not only cover suffrage but can comprise political participation in different forms. When problematising citizenship, it is valuable to have these inherent differing and sometimes conflicting normative ideas in mind, even if the aim would solely be for an empirical and not a normative or theoretical analysis.

As argued by Lister (2007; also by other scholars, c.f. Kymlicka, 1995), citizenship can be distinguished into two parts: citizenship as a status and as a practice. Status is about being a citizen; practice is about acting as a citizen as well as how citizenship is crafted and practised by other actors (Nedlund & Nordh, 2017), either, for example, actors working in welfare institutions or other citizens living in the same neighbourhood. To be a citizen means to enjoy the

rights of citizenship that are necessary for agency and social and political participation. Furthermore, to act as a citizen is to realize the full potential of that status.
Also, in parallel to what Wiener (1998) pointed out, the dimension of rights
cannot alone illustrate *how* citizenship is for citizens living with dementia. As a
'fulfilled member' of a community, citizenship also requires participation in one
way or another. These aspects are covered in the two other dimensions.

Access (to participation and justice)

The second dimension, *access,* concerns the conditions for practice citizenship
and sheds light on the relationship between citizens and the political and social
community. As Wiener (1998) points out, in order to understand the meaning
of citizenship it is necessary to study access to participation within the community. Political participation is central from a democratic perspective and is regulated in a variety of policies carried out by authoritative institutions. Access to
participation can be refused to individuals who are not in a position to practise
their citizenship rights, depending on factors such as lack of education or communications difficulties. By this, access relates to two different aspects: the formal, which is related to the legal–formal access to citizenship; and the
informal–substantial, which is often expressed in terms of inclusion and exclusion and can, for example, consist of access to social services and by that being
included in practice to social citizenship. In other words, citizenship is more than
merely the formal rights. Accordingly, formal rights might be settled but access
to political participation might be denied to individuals who cannot argue their
right to the informal parts of citizenship. We would like to extend this scope on
access to participation to also include access to social justice, or fairness.

As Wiener emphasises, if the formal aspect of citizenship is achieved, then it
is necessary to follow up and see how the practical implications of, or reasons
behind, the informal parts are achieved. People who do not have the possibility
to influence politics, policies or the actual situation, as, for example, in a care
setting, and do not have access to entitlements that they formally have a right
to claim, put under question the fundamental part of a democracy and a welfare system. This is not least because this access can be denied to people who
are not in a position to use their citizen rights. The dimension of access is essential in the concept of citizenship and thus important to study, analyse and problematise. Hence, the dimension of access concerns practical conditions for
participation and influence as well as insights into the process of deciding what
citizenship and its content (as in access to services) will be. An example of when
people living with dementia might be denied access to services, and thus dis-
criminated against, is if they also have a chronic hip disease. In a study of such
a situation, the conceptualisation of having a cognitive impairment and having
a hip disease in an evidence-based culture implied limited access to surgical

services (Graham, 2004). Thus, as the author of the study argues, this discrimination and denial of access violates the promotion of health-related citizenship rights of cognitively impaired individuals such as people living with dementia. Access is related to the criteria for citizenship practice. It also encompasses what is called 'the active citizenship', which encourages activeness in all forms – not least as active participation. This can be problematic for people with cognitive difficulties such as people living with dementia.

According to Lister (2007, 2009), political agency and political activism are important for citizenship from the perspective of their impact on both the wider community and the individuals involved. Political agency and activism are important for the wider community by allowing individuals to defend and extend the rights shared by other community members and to promote social capital and are important for individuals because involvement in a collective action can boost individuals and make them see themselves as political actors and citizens (Lister, 2007). This can, in the longer run, open formal politics to take into consideration the informal spheres of citizenship, such as the process of negotiation with welfare institutions and informal neighbourhood politics. By this, the informal spheres shed light on areas where, for example, women and people with dementia are visible, as a contrast to formal political systems in which they are underrepresented (Lister, 2009).

Access to justice is about seeking and obtaining a remedy to an intolerable situation through use of formal or informal institutions of justice and in conformity with human rights standards. As such, the process of accessing justice is inextricably linked to the idea of citizenship in and as practice. Take for example, the case of Manuela Sykes – a woman with dementia who at the time of the case was 89 years old and living in a care home. In February 2014, Ms Sykes won the right to return to her flat on a one-month trial basis after a court protection heard she was miserable in a care home. Unusually, the judge ruled that she could be named in media reports, in line with her wishes and because doing so was in the public interest. The case involved Manuela Sykes' liberty, residence and care, and for us, shows how citizenship simultaneously entails both internal and external processes.

The case of Manuela Sykes is unusual, though, not only because the judge authorised the revealing of her identity but also because most people with dementia have neither the resources nor the leverage to access justice in the way this wealthy former politician has done. This is not to detract from this act of citizenship but to highlight how there is often a wide gap between the principle of equal justice and its practice (Rhode, 2004). For example, during fieldwork undertaken by Bartlett for her PhD study on social exclusion in care homes, a woman told her that her husband had put her in the care home and so she wanted a divorce. She said it a few times. However, no one took her seriously or followed up. She had a voice but it did not count. In this case, citizenship was not enabled or practised. Accordingly, legal and social rights dissipate when someone has dementia and is in a care home.

Belonging (to what)

The third dimension concerns the citizens' *belonging* to a political entity or a community. We would elaborate on this element by asking 'what is it the people are belonging to?' or 'what is it that some people are not belonging to, i.e. excluded from?', 'why is it like that?' and 'how?'. Traditionally, belonging is based on nationality and is thus related to legal relations to a sovereign state that has been defined through jurisdiction of land or blood. The relations between the citizen and the community have been strengthened by the use of political symbolism, myths and languages. These perspectives define a kind of belonging that support a legally decided and cultural form of citizenship. Belonging relates to aspects of identity and processes of inclusion and exclusion, in other words, the difference and the tension between 'we' and 'them'. Citizenship is always exclusive; it has both an inclusionary and an exclusionary character. This does not have to be in terms of nationality but can also be in terms of being excluded from rights and duties or from social and cultural settings. Belonging to a community can take different forms, for example being regarded as an independent adult or as a person with his or her own experiences. Belonging is never fixed but continuously tested, which reflects the changed patterns of identity. Belonging tangents to normative ideas and discussion on equality versus difference. Equality relates to universalism, where every citizen has the possibility to participate as equal parts in the public sphere. Difference relates to particularism, which regard the differences of the citizens. A suggested compromise is to open up for differentiated pluralism (Siim, 2000; Lister, 2009) that aims to take both of these ideas into account. The continuous reconstruction of who belongs challenges formal rights as well as the state's role of protecting these rights. Citizenship also has a subjective side, which concerns the feeling and experience of oneself as a citizen in collective terms, that is, when you share the same experiences within a community and feel and experience that you belong (Bosniak, 2006; Siim, 2000; Yuval-Davies, 2011). Further, we also must recognise that there are shifts in understandings and experiences on where one belongs and what one identifies with. Belonging also relates to aspects such as solidarity to others and politics of recognition (c.f. Bosniak, 2006). The feeling of belonging can be shaped by previously drawn boundaries and is thus related not only to rights but also to how access to participation has been shaped in different settings; it is related to social categorisations, practices and relations (c.f. Nedlund & Nordh, 2017). Hence, belonging relates also to the 'actual political practices' that are connected to this membership of being a citizen (Wiener, 1998).

In other words, the third dimension, belonging, is not only regulated in the constitution but also constructed and practised by the citizens themselves in terms of identity, social positioning and institutional practices. Hence, belonging is closely linked to access. Both dimensions concern the practical possibilities to participate and influence politics and policy (Wiener, 1998) but also what becomes a citizenship content, as in the everyday actions and practices as a citizen and for example policy practice by people working in the welfare institutions. Both can be revealed discursively in policy documents. In the case of people living with dementia, this can concern, for example, participation in decisions that concern their own life situation.

Rights constitute the formal dimension, as access and belonging constitute the substantial dimensions. The dimension of rights does not alone provide sufficient information to understand citizenship in terms of being a fulfilled member of a community. Fulfilled citizenship also requires participation and practice in some way (Wiener, 1998, p. 26f) to recognise the voice of and respond to the citizen in need.

Citizenship-in-and-as-practice

According to Wiener (1998, 2013), citizenship practice is the process that constitutes the institutionalised terms of citizenship within a community, formed by principles of justice, the adherence to formal political and legal procedures, and norms and values in the society. As a generic concept, citizenship is not limited to a universal principle defining the rights and duties of individuals within a political community. As a practice, it is also an organizing principle of constitutional communities. As Wiener points out (2013), a practice approach to citizenship, which focuses on constitutional quality from a bottom-up perspective, enables thinking along the lines of the 'universalism of the particular'. Accordingly, citizenship practice forms the relation between the citizens and the community, that is, the procedures of participation as well as the day-to-day practices of citizen participation within a defined community. This implies that both the liberal and the communitarian and republican ideas can empirically take place at the same time, as can other normative ideas on what citizenship should embrace. The practices of citizenship – citizenship-in-and-as-practice – both in a policy context and in everyday situations are formed by this institutionalising process.

However, citizenship is a complex and contentious concept; various researchers and practitioners have different meanings of what citizenship encompasses and what citizenship should be. Citizenship is also a contextual concept; that is, the concept varies according to the social, political and cultural contexts and is also linked to individual experiences of citizenship. Citizenship is changeable and dynamic; it is constructed, created and given meaning. In this way, citizenship has both a formal side and a substantial side. That is, as citizens, we can formally have equal rights, but in practice we have various possibilities to use and enjoy them.

Citizenship can also be seen as a process and not just as a static form of status (e.g. being Swedish, being a Londoner, etc.) and results (in the form of e.g. rights and obligations but also services and support such as social care and health care). This process creates the inception of citizenship, that is, what could be called a citizenship process. In this process, various types of social representations are important when problematic descriptions and depictions of various citizens in policies and programmes become established (such as the portrayal of people with dementia that is ascribed in governing official policy documents).

The social representations also have practical implications in citizens' everyday life because they provide signals about how citizens perceive each other and also themselves (e.g. I am someone who should have something to say in this question). To regard citizenship as a process, something that is ongoing and constructed, also gives room to draw attention to matters of injustice, inequality and social exclusion, and to show that the formal rights do not – in practice – apply to all. Through this, we can observe how standards can stigmatize and discriminate and how attributions, understandings of power and social practices continuously are recreated. As such, citizenship is also interrelated, relational and transformative (Nedlund & Nordh, 2017). By having this perspective on citizenship, one can note that citizens are not passive recipients of aid and efforts without having an agency, that is, the human capacity to act, both individually and collectively, and – not least – highlighting that they, as citizens, are members of society.

For people with dementia, such a picture is more permissive and stands in contrast to the image of people with dementia as victims of their disease. Linking citizenship to agency also provides a space to see citizens as individual people with different social representations, social categories and identities. That is, in the social category of 'people with dementia' there is a variety of people with different social representations and belongings. Citizenship can by its focus on agency highlight the citizen's right to have the opportunity to participate, to be involved and to have influence in issues concerning daily life. It may be to have the agency as an individual or as a collective. Living with dementia can imply having agency with limitations, because people with dementia may need help and support from the welfare system. But this need does not have to stand in contrast to being recognized and regarded as an individual person with rights and also as an actor in society. Rather it is the joint recognition of being a person and an agent that still can be vulnerable.

As Wiener points out (1997, p. 10), by studying the relational dimension of citizenship and by regarding the dynamic role of citizenship, the universal principle of equality among all citizens and the particularistic reality of the persisting inequality among individuals that reside within one community come within the focus. Thus we can study citizenship practice as the politics and policies that deal with this tension and its impact on the organisational and philosophical task of accommodating diversity. The larger sociocultural context plays a role, as values, norms and beliefs influence how one perceives experiences and responds to the illness (O'Connor et al., 2007; Innes et al., 2004; Nedlund & Nordh, 2015; Nedlund & Nordh, 2017). 'The performance and behaviour of person with dementia are not exclusively determined by neuropathology but are also influenced by personal histories, social interactions and social context' (O'Connor et al., 2007, p. 56).

Diversity, and also not only the disease

The framework gives room for intersectionality, since people rarely, or rather never, have only dementia, but can also be categorised into other groups. This makes it possible to see if the citizenship practice for people with dementia is fragmented.

Citizenship as practice and citizenship in practice encompass the processes that contribute to institutionalize the terms of citizenship (Wiener, 1997, p. 598). The analysis of citizenship based on the concept of citizenship practice does not begin from an approach that defines citizenship legally according to citizenship rights. Instead, it aims at an understanding of characteristic features of citizenship, in this case for people with dementia, and assumes:

> citizenship to be constructed in practice particular to time, place, actors and institutions. It seeks to identify citizenship in its own context. (Wiener, 1997, p. 536)

Citizenship is the link between individual human agency and collective action. It also relates to the civil society.

The emerging discourse of people with dementia from a citizenship perspective

Studying and problematising dementia and situations for people living with a dementia diagnosis from a citizenship perspective have received increasing attention during the last decade. A great part of this interest started after Bartlett and O'Connor's article (2007), in which they presented their ideas of using a citizenship perspective to attain a more coherent understanding of research on dementia. Such point of departure implies that people with dementia are to be regarded, like other citizens, as equals with rights (and obligations). In research on dementia, this citizenship discourse can be regarded as a fourth turn: from dementia being regarded as a sign of aging, to a biomedical turn emphasising the medical conditions and the losses of agency and self in which people with dementia are depicted as 'demented patients', 'victims' (c.f. Fontana & Smith, 1989) or 'zombies' (Kessler, 2007), to the 'personhood turn' that focuses on seeing the person beyond the medical condition and in which dementia is regarded as a unique personal experience of living with dementia within broader social practices. This discourse focused on people's experiences of living with dementia (e.g. Aminzadeh et al., 2009), family members' experiences (e.g. Lyman, 1989), identity changes and the relationship to close relatives (e.g. Hydén & Nilsson, 2013) and communication patterns (e.g. Plejert et al., 2014). Furthermore, in their work, Bartlett and O'Connor (2007, 2010) also critically argued that to study people with dementia from a citizenship perspective implies to broaden the perspective from seeing only the person's individual experiences to also regarding the person as an actor in the society. A citizenship perspective implies, according to Bartlett and O'Connor, a kind of empowerment for people with dementia that emphasises individuals' possibility to be independent, the ability to formulate their own goals and to have power over their own lives.

With a citizenship discourse, the focus becomes to explore other types of arrangements in terms of enabling the various sociopolitical aspects of being a citizen and practising citizenship within a community. Even if research before Bartlett and O'Connor's pioneering work, or research not departing from this fourth turn, has to some smaller extent elaborated on people with dementia as citizens, commonly by analysing capacity to vote in elections (c.f. Karlawish et al., 2004; McEldowney & Teaster, 2009; Wislowski & Cuellar, 2006) or setting dementia in a social, political and legal context (c.f. Barnes & Brannelly, 2008; Boller & Forbes, 1998; Innes, 2002), the notion of citizenship was not explicitly applied.

An increasing body of research critically problematises citizenship and social exclusion of people with dementia, to challenge an existing understanding that people with dementia are incapable of participating in social interactions (c.f. Baldwin, 2008; Behuniak, 2010, 2011; Brannelly, 2011; Gilmour & Brannelly, 2009; Kelly & Innes, 2013; Wilkinson, 2001). Other studies shed light on citizenship from a legal perspective related to aspects of self-determination (c.f. Boyle, 2008, 2010; Nedlund & Taghizadeh Larsson, 2016). Another type of problematization is how citizenship can be practised through self-help groups, by advocacies and by people living with dementia as active co-researchers (Bartlett, 2014). Studies have also problematized the institutional meetings between care managers and people with dementia from a citizenship perspective (Nordh & Nedlund, 2016; Taghizadeh Larsson & Österholm, 2014). Few studies seek to problematise and conceptualise citizenship practice by the role of policies in order to increase the understanding of how policy narratives have constructed people with dementia as policy targets and service users, and the further implications on claiming citizenship (Baldwin, 2013; Nedlund & Nordh, 2015, 2017). Also, from a feminist citizenship perspective, one study has explored gender differences in relation to dementia care in order to inform policy and future research to address inequalities and promote citizenship (Bartlett et al., 2016).

What Bartlett and O'Connor (2007) also suggest for further research on citizenship and dementia is to regard citizenship as practice, that is, to understand citizenship as 'something individuals achieve for themselves, through the power dynamics of everyday talk and practice' (2007, p. 109). Other researchers have also offered ways to conceptualise this approach, such as Gilmour and Brannelly (2009; also Barnes & Brannelly, 2008; Brannelly, 2011a, 2011b), who, relying on ethics of care, argue for inclusionary practices such as involving older people in the design of services that have a direct benefit in citizenship terms. By that, citizenship practice is regarded more in terms of facilitating participation and support and sustaining citizenship of people through practice, for example through relational caring (Brannelly, 2011). Another way of understanding citizenship as practice has been presented by Baldwin (2008), in terms of narratives. Citizenship practice has also been conceptualized by Nedlund and Nordh (2015, 2017), who draw on elements of policy narratives to reveal the important aspect of power in order to participate and influence the shaping of policies and the crafting of citizens and the space in which citizenship is continuously practised. Citizenship practice has guided and been explored in empirical research (c.f. Clarke & Bailey, 2016; Dupuis et al., 2016; Österholm & Hydén, 2016; Wiersma et al., 2016), also in terms of the importance of neighbourhood in being and acting citizenship practice for people with dementia (Phinney et al., 2016; Ward et al., 2016).

These examples show the importance of studying citizenship practice. However, there still is a need to problematise why citizenship is a useful point of departure for exploring life with dementia and how citizenship in and as practice can be enabled. This is what we have aimed to elaborate further and to present a way of understanding and approaching citizenship practice for people with dementia.

Enabling citizenship in and as practice for people living with dementia

Having outlined key definitional features of citizenship, in this section we consider how citizenship is or can be practised in a policy context as well as in everyday practices. The tension between the three elements – rights, access and belonging – sheds light on the different and unequal possibilities to take apart and formulate the description of a problem (Wiener, 1998). One way of examining this tension is to return to the quote by Jim Mann at the beginning of the chapter about 'assuming one's place at the table', where the table could be construed as a space for citizenship. The citizenship space takes place in a specific institutional context where institutionalised norms influence discourse and interpreted borders on the meaning of citizenship (for the citizen in concern). This meaning can differ from one citizen group to another. In other words, the table is placed in a particular social context that could concern topics ranging from macro-level political decisions to a micro-level decision affecting a person's everyday life. What is regarded as a space for citizenship is not once and for all stated but may be re-defined.

Relations between citizens are not fixed; rather they are fluid and open to interpretation and reinterpretation. So, when thinking about spaces and places for citizenship, and in particular, who is assumed to belong around a table, it is our places in the social hierarchies and what power and influence they can wield that will help to determine the outcome of such struggles (Lister, 2009). However, as Colebatch (2011) points out, it is also important to ask 'who is sitting around the table' because this shapes the agenda, and in this case, how citizenship is practised. There are, therefore, several questions to ask about power relations before citizenship can be enabled. First, as presented above, how the meaning of citizenship is understood depends on who is participating and not participating and on who is regarded as belonging (being included) or excluded from the deliberations at the table. Power thus relates to the way the phenomenon, in this case citizenship, becomes understood. A change in how citizenship can be understood can be described as a 'paradigmatic change' (Hall, 1993). The tension between rights, access and belonging also sheds light on the possibilities to claim rights and further to formulate what will temporarily be understood as a policy problem. As also pointed out by Wiener, citizenship is thus a product of a collective changeable description of problems that must be visible to be established. Citizenship can therefore be regarded as a product of a collective and ever-changing description of social problems in which a social phenomenon becomes established and visible. When a phenomenon appears as invisible or unproblematic, one can understand it as a result of forgotten questioning and strong forms of answering and vice versa (Nedlund & Nordh, 2017; Turnbull, 2013). In the context of people with dementia, citizenship for people with dementia has started to be studied – in terms of rights, access and belonging – which is also illustrated by Jim Mann's quotation as well as Rose Kornfeld Matte's quotation. In other words, the way in which a phenomenon gets attention, and the underlying power relations linked to it as well as the practice, are defining the characteristics of citizenship. Furthermore, this also depends on who is allowed to participate in the collective, and in the particular institutional context, in this case the space for citizenship, and further, by whom someone is allowed. As Wiener points out:

> Citizens contribute to the creation of a community, yet not all persons who reside within the same geographical space enjoy the same citizenship privileges. This is where the tension lies. (Wiener, 1997, p. 534)

In other words, citizenship is exclusionary. It relates to the distribution of power among actors. Citizenship – being and acting as a citizen – is very much about participating and being involved in society and in decisions that concern everyday life. It can include participating in and influencing policies, such as the goals and visions that should be in the community, and participating in decisions concerning one's own everyday life, as in, for example, access to services. But it is important that this is done on one's own terms and based on one's own conditions, not least in regard to an individual's own ability to formulate goals and to enable the individual to have power over his or her own life. This needs to be in terms not only of how to protect people's right to self-determination but also of how to support people in making decisions and exercising their citizenship (Nedlund & Taghizadeh Larsson, 2016). This is also within the responsibility of other citizens.

Citizenship as a status and citizenship as a practice are not once and for all defined but are dynamic and continuously contested and re-constructed over time. The asymmetry and variability can be analysed and problematised by the use of the three elements: rights, access and belonging. These different elements might sometimes be intertwined but on other occasions will be fragmented, thus having different implications for the citizens concerned.

What about the obligations of being and acting as an active citizen? The idea of active citizenship by having access to participation to enjoy access to justice may create expectations of and excessive demands on people with dementia. There is a strong expectation that citizens are autonomous and self-determinant and that everyone should be able to understand their own situation and make independent decisions. Sometimes it may be difficult for people with dementia to live up to these demands and expectations. This is also a reason it is important to use a citizenship perspective to explore the different inclusive ways of how citizenship can be enabled for people living with dementia. Citizenship is something interrelated between citizens in terms of solidarity, where some citizens agree to step back to benefit others with greater needs (Nedlund & Nordh, 2017).

By this we can enable a view of people with dementia not as pathological but rather as people who belong to a social and political context in which they interact with others. People with dementia can be regarded as having a status and as having agency and also can exercise rights (also through substitute decision-makers).

This view presents the possibility that persons with dementia actually will make use of their cognitive and communicative abilities; that other persons will support these abilities in everyday interaction; and that new understandings of the person with dementia can be introduced and used in research, policy contexts and education. This is what assuming one's place around the table is about and it clearly relates to rights, access and belonging and thus to citizenship-in-and-as-practice.

References

Aminzadeh, F., Dalziel, W. B., Molnar, F. J. & Garcia, L. J. (2009). Symbolic meaning of relocation to a residential care facility for persons with dementia. *Aging and Mental Health, 13,* 487–496.

Baldwin, C. (2008). Narrative, citizenship and dementia: The personal and the political. *Journal of Aging Studies, 22,* 222–228.

Baldwin, C. (2013). *Narrative social work: Theory and application.* Bristol: Policy Press.

Barnes, M. & Brannelly, T. (2008). Achieving care and social justice for people with dementia. *Nursing Ethics, 15,* 384–395.

Barnes, C. & Mercer, G. (2003). *Disability (Key Concepts).* Cambridge, UK: Policy Press.

Bartlett, R. & O'Connor, D. (2007). From personhood to citizenship: Broadening the lens for dementia practice and research. *Journal of Aging Studies, 21,* 107–118.

Bartlett, R. & O'Connor, D. (2010). *Broadening the Dementia Debate: Towards Social Citizenship.* Bristol: Policy Press.

Bartlett, R. (2014). Citizenship in action: The lived experience of citizens with dementia who campaign for social change. *Disability & Society, 29,* 1291–1304.

Bartlett, R., Gjernes, T., Lotherington, A.-T. & Obstefelder, A. (2016). Gender, citizenship and dementia care: A scoping review of studies to inform policy and future research. *Health and Social Care in the Community.* doi:10.1111/hsc.12340

Behuniak, S. M. (2010). Toward a political model of dementia: Power as compassionate care. *Journal of Aging Studies, 24,* 231–240.

Behuniak, S. M. (2011). The living dead? The construction of people with Alzheimer's disease as zombies. *Aging and Society, 31,* 70–92.

Boller, B. & Forbes, M. (1998). History of dementia and dementia in history: An overview. *Journal of Neurological Sciences. 158(2),* 125–133.

Boyle, G. (2008). The Mental Capacity Act 2005: Promoting the citizenship of people with dementia? *Health and Social Care in the Community, 16,* 529–537.

Boyle, G. (2010). Social policy for people with dementia in England: Promoting human rights? *Health and Social Care in the Community, 18,* 511–519.

Boyle, G. (2014). Social policy for people with dementia in England: Promoting human rights? *Health and Social Care in the Community, 18,* 511–519.

Bosniak, Linda. (2006). *The Citizen and the Alien – Dilemmas of Contemporary Membership.* Princeton, NJ: Princeton University Press.

Brannelly, T. (2011a). Sustaining citizenship: People with dementia and the phenomenon of social death. *Nursing Ethics, 18,* 662–671.

Brannelly, T. (2011b). That others matter: The moral achievement – Care ethics and citizenship in practice with people with dementia. *Ethics and Social Welfare, 5,* 210–216.

Colebatch, H. (2011). Challenge and development: The emerging understanding of policy work. *Politika misao, 48,* 11–24.

Clarke, C. & Bailey, C. (2016). Narrative citizenship, resilience and inclusion with dementia: On the inside or on the outside of physical and social places. *Dementia, 15,* 434–452.

Dupuis, S., Kontos, P., Mitchell, M., Jonas-Simpson, C. & Gray, J. (2016). Re-claiming citizenship through the arts. *Dementia, 15,* 358–380.

Dwyer, P. (2010). *Understanding Social Citizenship: Themes and Perspectives for Policy and Practice* (2nd ed.) Bristol: Policy Press.

Fontana, A. & Smith, R. W. (1989). Alzheimer's disease victims: The 'unbecoming' of self and the normalization of competence. *Sociological Perspectives, 32*, 35–46.

Graham, R. (2004). Cognitive citizenship: Access to hip surgery for people with dementia. *Health, 8*, 295–310.

Gilmour, J. A. & Brannelly, T. (2009). Representations of people with dementia – Subaltern, person, citizen. *Nursing Inquiry, 17*, 240–247.

Hafford-Letchfield, T., Couchman, W., Leonard, K., Woods, S., Avery, P. & Webster, M. (2010). Developing learning materials to promote positive interaction with people with dementia: We are all in it together! In XVII ISA World Congress of Sociology, 13 July 2010, Gothenburg, Sweden.

Hakosalo, H. (2011). A powerful precedent: The recognition of women's academic rights (1901) and the 1906 parliamentary reform in Finland. In L. Freidenvall & J. Rönnbäck (Eds.), *Bortom Rösträtten: Kön, politik och medborgarskap i Norden*. Stockholm: Samtidshistoriska institutet.

Hall, P. (1993). Policy paradigms, social learning, and the state: The case of economic policymaking in Britain. *Comparative Politics, 25*, 275–296.

Hydén, L. C. & Nilsson, E. (2013). Couples with dementia: Positioning the 'we'. *Dementia, 14*, 716–733.

Innes, A. (2002). The social and political context of formal dementia care provision. *Ageing & Society, 22*, 483–499.

Innes, A., Archibald, C. & Murphy, C. (Eds.) (2004). *Dementia and Social Inclusion: Marginalised Groups and Marginalised Areas of Dementia Research, Care and Practice*. London: Jessica Kingsley.

Isin, E. & Turner, B. S. (2007). Investigating citizenship: An agenda for citizenship studies. *Citizenship Studies, 11*, 5–17.

Joppke, C. (2007). Transformation of citizenship: Status, rights, identity. *Citizenship Studies, 11*, 37–48.

Mann, J. (2015). Claiming full citizenship: Self-determination, personalization, individualized funding. In [Conference Brochure] 2015 International Conference, October 15–October 17, 2015, The Hyatt Regency, Vancouver, Canada. Retrieved from http://interprofessional.ubc.ca/ClaimingFullCitizenship2015/brochure.pdf, 5 May 2016.

Karlawish, J. et al. (2004). Addressing the ethical, legal, and social issues raised by voting by persons with dementia. *Journal of the American Medical Association, 292*, 1345–1350.

Kelly, F. & Innes, A. (2013). Human rights, citizenship and dementia care nursing. *International Journal of Older People Nursing, 8*, 61–70.

Kessler, L. (2007). *Dancing with Rose: Finding Life in the Land of Alzheimer's*. New York: Viking Press.

Kornfeld-Matte, R. (2015). Statement of the independent expert on the enjoyment of all human rights by older person. In First WHO Ministerial Conference on Global Action Against Dementia. Geneva, Switzerland: United Nations Human Rights: Office of the High Commissioner for Human Rights. Retrieved from www.ohchr.org/EN/Issues/OlderPersons/IE/Pages/IEOlderPersons.aspx, March 13, 2017.

Kymlicka, W. (1995). *Multicultural Citizenship: A Liberal Theory of Minority Rights*. Oxford: Oxford University Press.

Kymlicka, W. & Patten, A. (Eds.) (2003). *Language Rights and Political Theory*. Oxford: Oxford University Press.

Lister, R. (2007). Inclusive citizenship: Realizing the potential. *Citizenship Studies, 11*, 49–61.

Lister, R. (2009). *Understanding Theories and Concepts in Social Policy*. Bristol: Policy Press.

Lyman, K. A. (1989). Bringing the social back in: A critique of the biomedicalization of dementia. *The Gerontologist, 29*, 597–605.

Marshall, T. H. (1991/1950). *Citizenship and Social Class*. Cambridge: Cambridge University Press.

McEldowney, R. & Teaster, P. B. (2009). Land of the free, home of the brave: Voting accommodations for older adults. *Journal of Aging & Social Policy, 21*, 159–171.

Mental Health Foundation (2015). *Dementia, rights, and the social model of disability A new direction for policy and practice?* Policy discussion paper.

Nedlund, A.-C. & Nordh, J. (2015). Crafting citizen(ship) for people with dementia: How policy narratives at national level in Sweden informed politics of time from 1975 to 2013. *Journal of Aging Studies, 34*, 123–133.

Nedlund, A.-C. & Nordh, J. (2017). Constructing citizens: A matter of labelling, imaging and underlying rationales in the case of people with dementia. *Critical Policy Studies*. doi.org/10.1080/19460171.2017.1297730. Accepted for publication.

Nedlund, A.-C. & Taghizadeh Larsson, A. (2016). To protect and to support: How citizenship and self-determination are legally constructed and managed in practice for people living with dementia in Sweden. *Dementia, 15*, 343–357.

Nordh, J. & Nedlund, A.-C. (2016). To co-ordinate information in practice: Dilemmas and strategies in care management for citizens with dementia. *Journal of Social Services Research*. doi: 10.1080/01488376.2016.1217580.

O'Connor, D., Phinney, A., Smith, A., Small, J., Purves, B., Perry, J., Drance, E., Donnelly, M., Chaudhury, H. & Beattie, L. (2007). Personhood in dementia care: Developing a research agenda for broadening the vision. *Dementia, 6*, 121–142.

Österholm, H. J. & Hydén, L. C. (2016). Citizenship as practice: Handling communication problems in encounters between persons with dementia and social workers. *Dementia*. doi: 10.1177/1471301214563959.

Phinney, A., Kelson, E., Baumbusch, J., O'Connor, D. & Purves, B. (2016). Walking in the neighbourhood: Performing social citizenship in dementia. *Dementia, 15*, 381–394.

Plejert, C., Jansson, G. & Yazdanpanah, M. (2014). Response practices in multilingual interaction with an older Persian woman in a Swedish residential home. *Journal of Cross-Cultural Gerontology, 29*, 1–23.

Rhode, D. (2004). *Access to Justice*. New York: Oxford University Press.

Richardson, D. (1998). Sexuality and citizenship. *Sociology, 32*, 83–100.

Shachar, A. (2014). Introduction: Citizenship and the 'right to have rights'. *Citizenship Studies, 18(2)*, 114–124.

Siim, B. (2000). *Gender and Citizenship: Politics and Agency in France, Britain and Denmark*. Cambridge: Cambridge University Press.

Taghizadeh Larsson, A. & Österholm, J. H. (2014). How are decisions on care services for people with dementia made and experienced? A systematic review and qualitative synthesis of recent empirical findings. *International Psychogeriatrics, 26*, 1849–1862.

Townsend, A. & Wilcock, A. (2004). Occupational justice and client-centred practice: A dialogue. *Canadian Journal of Occupational Therapy, 71(2)*, 75–87.

Turnbull, N. (2013). The questioning theory of policy practice: Outline of an integrated analytical framework. *Critical Policy Studies, 7*, 115–131.

Van der Ploeg, E., Eppingstall, B. & O'Connor, D. (2016). Internet video chat (Skype) family conversations as a treatment of agitation in nursing home residents with dementia. *International Psychogeriatrics, 28(4)*, 697–698.

Ward, R., Campbell, S. & Keady, J. (2016). 'Gonna make yer gorgeous': Everyday transformation, resistance and belonging in the care-based hair salon. *Dementia, 15*, 395–413.

Wiener, A. (1998). *'European' Citizenship Practice: Building Institutions of a Non-state*. Boulder, CO: Westview.

Wiener, A. (2013). Toward global citizenship practice? In X. Guillaume & J. Huysmans (Eds.), *Citizenship and Security: The Constitution of Political Being*. Abingdon: Routledge.

Wiener, A. & Della Salla, V. (1997). Constitution-making and citizenship practice – Bridging the democracy gap in the EU? *Journal of Common Market Studies, 35*, 596–614.

Wiersma, E. C., O'Connor, D. L., Loiselle, L., Hickman, K., Heibein, B., Hounam, B. & Mann, J. (2016). Creating space for citizenship: The impact of group structure on validating the voices of people with dementia. *Dementia, 15*, 414–433.

Wilkinson, H. (2001). Empowerment and decision-making for people with dementia: The use of legal interventions in Scotland. *Aging & Mental Health, 5*, 322–328.

Wislowski, A. & Cuellar, N. (2006). Voting rights for older Americans with dementia: Implications for health care providers. *Nursing Outlook, 54*, 68–73.

Yuval-Davis, N. (2011). *The Politics of Belonging: Intersectional Contestations*. Los Angeles: Sage.

5

PATHWAYS WITHIN DEMENTIA DIAGNOSIS

Charlotta Plejert, Danielle Jones and Elizabeth Peel

Introduction

In this chapter, we foreground different dementia diagnostic pathways across three temporal phases of the process of diagnosis: from initial history-taking in memory clinic assessment to the disclosure and discussion of diagnosis. Therefore, we are interested in not only pathways *to* a diagnosis of dementia but also the pathways and experiences *within* the diagnostic process, exploring the interactions that occur during this process. Specifically, we focus first on conversational profiling and differential diagnosis during memory clinic assessment; second on interpreter-mediated dementia evaluations; and third on disclosure and discussion of diagnosis.

A dementia diagnosis is a life-changing and often overwhelming experience, both for the person who receives the diagnosis and for relatives and other close people. For some, however, getting a diagnosis may also be a relief, because it offers an explanation for worrying symptoms. Pathways towards a diagnosis, however, vary a great deal from person to person and family to family. In Western societies at least, with growing cultural awareness of dementias, public health campaigns, and heightened media profile (Peel, 2014), increasing numbers of people and their families are seeking a formal dementia diagnosis. In the early stages, signs such as mild forgetfulness and other cognitive and behavioural changes may be thought of as indicators of stress or depression or caused by factors other than a dementia disease. It might also be the case that the person with dementia is not able to self-monitor and therefore perceives symptoms of the disease differently than do family and friends. This may also affect help-seeking behaviours. In addition, various cultural belief-systems affect if, when and to what extent people turn to health-care services. Whereas most people in cultures influenced by a biomedical perspective view dementia as an illness, there are also groups and populations that treat dementia symptoms as a result of many things, including natural signs of aging, madness or even enlightenment (e.g. Dilworth-Anderson & Gibson, 2002; Leibing & Cohen, 2006). Some studies have observed differences between populations (in the United States) concerning the duration from the point of first notice and symptom recognition to final diagnosis, suggesting that people of a certain ethnicity, for example African-American and Hispanic people, have a longer lag time between first notice and diagnosis than do white Americans (e.g. Schrauf & Iris, 2011). An explanation for this difference might be reflected in how families choose to deal with symptoms. In the study by Schrauf and Iris (2011), it was claimed that Hispanic and African American caregivers 'effectively provide a kind of "scaffolding" for the patient' (p. 743), which was a way of actively dealing with the disease, but also affected the length of time before seeking medical attention. This potentially also explains why, for example, African Americans show greater symptom severity at the time of diagnosis than some other populations (Dilworth-Anderson et al., 2002; Shadlen et al., 1999).

In addition to issues related to ethnicity, several other sociocultural influences inform people's understanding and experience of diagnosis, for example gender (Erol et al., 2015), sexual identity (Peel & McDaid, 2015), age (Rosser et al., 2010) and social class (O'Connor et al., 1991). There is also geographical variability in dementia service provision, both nationally and internationally, which impacts both access to and the experience of services and adequate care. Differences in diagnostic procedures may also vary, for example whether diagnostic testing occurs in primary or secondary care or whether pre-diagnostic counselling and post-diagnostic support is offered. These modes of service delivery and structural health provision issues make a difference in terms of referral rates to access further testing, the time people have to wait to access memory services and likely their experience of the process.

Once a person who is suspected to have a dementia disease seeks care, she or he will undergo dementia assessment. The diagnostic process comprises numerous different parts, ordinarily consisting of a combination of history-taking (medical interview), formal tests of cognitive functioning, physical and psychiatric examinations, and ancillary investigations, blood tests, brain scans and lumbar punctures. Sometimes further investigations may be needed, such as extended neuropsychological testing, particularly if screening tests are normal or equivocal, and there is still a concern about cognitive and behavioural changes (Adelman & Daly, 2005).

The processes involved in a dementia evaluation are of great importance in several ways. It is not just a matter of reaching an accurate diagnosis, but the actual practices that occur between clinicians, patients and patients' companions are key for how pathways within dementia diagnosis are experienced. Patient satisfaction with the diagnostic process must be achieved. Building an enabling and trusting relationship with the clinicians in charge of the evaluations is an important part of turning an already challenging situation into something less emotionally taxing, especially as patients and carers view the diagnostic process as labyrinthine (Samsi et al., 2014) and (similarly) subsequent access to services as akin to navigating a maze (Peel & Harding, 2014).

Research on dementia diagnostic practices has so far primarily been carried out within the field of medicine. More recently, however, it has become a focus in social scientific research, particularly that which examines what happens in patient–doctor encounters. To date, this line of research has explored, for example, how people talk about their symptoms and how the occurrence of specific interactional features can be used to assist in the diagnosis of memory complaints (Elsey et al., 2015; Jones et al., 2016) and how a diagnosis is delivered and received (c.f. Heritage & Maynard, 2006; Lecouturier et al., 2008; Maynard & Frankel, 2006). Recent research has also highlighted specific aspects of dementia evaluations for ethnic minority patients, where an interpreter is needed in order to mediate talk between clinical staff and patients and their companions (Plejert et al., 2015; Majlesi & Plejert, 2016). It is through a social scientific lens that we approach the pathways within dementia diagnosis that are the focus of this chapter.

Conversation analysis

One way of understanding the processes involved in dementia diagnosis is to study the practices and actions that are established in, and through, interaction between the participants at hand. For this purpose, the framework of Conversation Analysis (CA) (e.g. Schegloff, 2007; Sidnell & Stivers, 2013) has proved useful, for the study not only of dementia (e.g. Chatwin, 2014) but also other conditions that affect language and interaction (e.g. Goodwin, 2003).

CA has its origin in sociology and ethnomethodology and is a theoretically and methodologically distinctive approach to the study of talk-in-interaction. The principle objective of CA is to discover the patterns, mechanisms and practices of interaction, which underlie our social competencies, by examining recorded instances of naturally occurring interactions. These recordings prove suitable for repeated examination and have revealed the cumulative empirical findings of the discipline, for example turn taking (Sacks et al., 1974), turn design (Drew, 2005), sequence organisation (Schegloff, 2007), repair (Schegloff et al., 1977) and social action (Schegloff, 1996). Today, video recordings serve as the basis for most analyses, since they provide access to both verbal and non-verbal features of interactions, which can be vital when investigating and understanding social conduct. CA has been applied successfully in a variety of primary and secondary medical services, exploring the features and practices within a range of medical communications. These studies have informed medical practice and have altered certain diagnostic processes (Heritage et al., 2007; Robson et al., 2012; Stivers, 2007). This way of feeding back into the areas under investigation is particularly typical for the branch commonly referred to as 'applied CA' (see Antaki, 2011). The three areas presented in the sections that follow may all be viewed as representative of this applied approach to CA.

Conversational profiling and differential diagnosis during memory clinic assessments

In many countries worldwide, there is an increase in the number of people referred to memory clinics and other specialist services. This is partially due to a raised awareness of the benefits of an early or 'timely' diagnosis (Brooker et al., 2014) for accessing health and social care interventions, enabling future care planning and increasing the efficacy of both drug and non-drug treatments. This development is also true for the United Kingdom, where referral rates are already high and expected to rise even further (Royal College of Psychiatrists, 2013). A problem that arises from this significant increase in patients referred to memory clinics is the pressure to provide both a speedy and an accurate diagnosis; this presents challenges for specialist practitioners. One specific difficulty is the need to distinguish dementia from other forms of psychological, cognitive or further memory problems that display similar symptomology, for example depression, trauma, mild cognitive impairment (MCI) and functional memory disorder (FMD). The differentiation between diagnoses relies on a lengthy evaluation process, meaning that it can be a difficult and time-consuming procedure. It may also be the case that test results are equivocal. Additional tools that could be used to assist in the diagnostic process are therefore needed, particularly if they could speed up the diagnostic process and decrease the need for complex further neuropsychological testing that can result in anxiety for patients. One relevant aspect of these concerns deals with how experienced clinicians often create a 'working diagnosis', formed on the basis of their initial impressions of the first few minutes of conversation with a patient with memory problems (Jones et al., 2016). The exact nature of this working diagnosis is of great interest for CA researchers, who have the tools for providing insights on how this diagnosis comes about and to what extent it is valid. Previous research on differentiating between epileptic and non-epileptic seizures suggests that analyses of how patients describe their problems (*what* they say or the content of their talk), for example using certain metaphors, as well as *how* they answer questions, may contain important information for their eventual diagnosis (e.g. Reuber et al., 2009; Plug et al., 2011) and may thus comprise elements that assist clinicians in distinguishing between different diagnoses. A similar approach has been used by Jones et al. (2016), who utilized CA methodology for differentiating between patients with neurodegenerative dementia and FMD.

The study by Jones et al. (2016) represents an initial analysis of data from a larger study using CA in the memory clinic to identify potential interactional and linguistic diagnostic pointers. Jones et al. (2016) present findings based on the analysis of a subset of 25 video and audio recordings of initial consultations between neurologists and patients referred to a specialist memory clinic in a UK city. Data were collected between 2012 and 2014. The patients were referred to the memory clinic through a variety of pathways, including from primary care general practice (GPs) or other secondary care services such as non-specialist neurology and psychiatry. A 'gold standard' clinical diagnosis was made by three consultant neurologists with a special interest in memory disorders on the basis of a patient's initial visit, including screening with the Addenbrooke's Cognitive Examination (ACE-R) and subsequent detailed neuropsychological test battery and magnetic resonance imaging (MRI) of the brain. Nine of the patients included received a diagnosis of a neurodegenerative memory disorder (average ACE-R score 56/100, range from 28 to 80) and 16 were diagnosed with FMD (average ACE-R score 93/100, range from 85 to 99) (for a definition of FMD see Blackburn et al., 2014). Sixteen of the patients were female and nine were male. The patients' ages ranged from 47 to 77 years. The initial history-taking phase of the encounters, which formed the basis of the analysis, lasted between 7 minutes and 28 seconds and 32 minutes and 29 seconds. None of the patients who ultimately received a diagnosis of a dementia attended the clinic alone, whereas 11 of the 16 patients with FMD came unaccompanied. Recordings were transcribed in considerable detail, using CA transcription conventions (Jefferson, 2004) and were analysed in accordance with CA methodology. Initial analyses revealed five interactional features that appeared relevant for the purpose of differentiating between dementia and FMD. These features were:

1 Patients' abilities to answer questions concerning personal information, for example their age or where they lived;

2 If patients were able to display functional working memory from within the interaction itself;

3 If patients were able to respond to compound questions;

4 The time taken to respond to questions; and

5 The level of specific details offered by patients when they gave accounts of their memory failure experiences.

Analyses of the first feature, responses to questions about personal information, revealed that people with FMD were able to produce answers quickly, unproblematically and accurately. In contrast, people with dementia displayed difficulties producing correct information, which could lead to repair-sequences in which the clinician or companion had to repeat or rephrase the questions or provide further explanatory information. For example, a question about age was promptly answered with no delay by a person with FMD, whereas a person with dementia might initiate repair, either as a result of not comprehending the question or confusing the question with something else, for example date of birth (cf. Jones et al., 2016, pp. 502–3).

Another interactional feature that aided the process of differentiating patients with FMD from people with dementia was the display of working memory in interaction. Examples from conversations during the history-taking part of the consultation demonstrated that people with FMD typically were able to display working memory in relation to what someone else had previously said in the consultation, for example in terms of remembering and answering prior questions. People with FMD were also able to recall and repeat information that they had previously mentioned themselves, often after a significant time had passed. These latter accounts were also often marked by phrases such as 'like I said' or 'as I say'. An example of this feature is illustrated in Excerpt 1, below. (Transcription conventions follow Jefferson (2004) and are found at the end of the chapter.)

Excerpt 1 (DOC=Doctor, PAT=Patient, OTH=Companion)

```
01   DOC: can I ask what other things?
02   PAT: .hhh stu:pid things, (.) stupid things.=if
03        .hh uhm say you've, (0.3) a- (.) admin at
04        work'll bring me a- or: can you ring
05        this pe:rson (.) and there's a phone number,
06        (0.2) it can take me up to ten times to be able
07        to, (0.2) get the phone number off the paper,
08        the correct number onto fo:rm.
09   ((7 minutes and 40 seconds omitted))
10   DOC: how are you with numbers an'(0.[2) arithm]etic,
11   PAT:                                 [terrible.]
12   PAT: t[errible.]
13   DOC: [has that]cha:nged?
14   PAT: .hh I've never been brilliant.=
15   OTH: =yeah.
16   PAT: >it's a-< it's always been a we:ak.=
17   OTH: =you've been more of a wor:dsmith
18        than a,(0.[4) than a: ]mathematician
19   PAT:           [y(h)es:. absolutely.]
20   OTH: sh[all we say.]
21   PAT:    [yes:, I ha]ve. .hh but, erm >like I say,<
22        e:ven: jus:t (.) cha- doing the phone number or:
23        sa- the slightest little things now I can't
24        seem to add up.
```

The doctor (line 01) is touching off a question based on the companion's previous assertion that 'other things' about the patient's memory had been pointed out to them as being problematic. The patient produces an example about her inability to accurately copy phone numbers as evidence of other memory problems she has experienced. Within the seven minutes omitted from the transcript the patient finishes this discussion about her problem with phone numbers, with her husband likening her difficulty to 'dyslexia'. The consultation then goes on to discuss several unrelated issues such as the patient's work, when the problems started, the anxiety the patient experiences and her spatial awareness. After this prolonged period of time, the neurologist asks how the patient is with numbers (line 10). After admitting to be 'terrible' (lines 11 and 12), and the companion acknowledging the patient's proficiency with words rather than numbers (lines 17 and 18), the patient again proceeds to use the example of her difficulty with phone numbers as evidence of how 'terrible' she is. Here the patient prefaces the repetition with 'like I say' (line 21), to mark her self-repetition and to display that she is aware that the information she is producing has already been given earlier. This interactional resource, which displays working memory, appears as a feature in the interactions with patients with FMD and contributes to their conversational profile. Unlike the patients with FMD, people with dementia were often unable to display memories during consultations in the way exemplified in Excerpt 1. In addition, in cases where people with dementia repeated themselves, they did not display any markers that demonstrated that they were aware of their repetitions (e.g. 'like I said'). Rather, repeated information was produced as if for the first time, something which has been demonstrated previously in CA work on interaction and dementia (Hydén et al., 2012; Jones, 2015).

The third interactional feature documented by Jones et al. (2016) concerned patients' abilities to respond to compound or 'multi-unit' questions (cf. Linell et al., 2003). This is a form of questioning that is very commonly used in institutional interaction, for example medical settings, court trials, police interrogations, etc. In relation to potential memory problems, multi-unit questions are demanding, since they require that a person remember several successive questions and provide answers to each one of them. In the Jones et al. study, people with FMD did not display any difficulties responding to multi-unit questions. In addition, they frequently also provided lengthy and detailed answers that covered what the clinician had asked about. People with dementia, however, demonstrated difficulties comprehending questions and also had problems recalling the different parts in their responses. Excerpt 2 provides an illustration of this feature.

Excerpt 2 (taken from Jones et al., 2016, p. 505)

```
01   DOC: .hh do you have any problems er with
02        reading or writing.
03        (0.6)
04   DOC: or spelling?
05        (1.2)
06   PAT: .hh er, (4.0) er, (0.2) tck what do you
```

```
07          mean, r-reading?
08   DOC: yeah. can you read OK?
09          (0.3)
10   PAT: yeah, I can read.
11   DOC: can you write what you want?
12   PAT: .hhh er, well it takes me a lot longer.
13          I have to sit and think about it.= er
14          when my pal's with me (0.5) he sometimes
15          b- b[etter with] what to do like.
16   DOC: [yeah.    ]
17          (1.4)
18   PAT: d'you know what I mean?
19   DOC: can you spell OK?
20          (0.2)
21   PAT: .hh rr, er, I'm n- not very good
22          speller.= but (0.4) sometimes, (1.4)
23          it- (1.0) an' it dun't come to me.
```

The patient does not accurately respond to all three parts of the multi-unit question (lines 01–04) and instead, after a lengthy inter-turn gap (line 05) and turn initial pause (line 06), seeks clarification from the doctor (lines 06 and 07). The doctor re-issues the questions individually, after which the patient responds. This exemplifies the difficulties people with dementia displayed in recalling and processing multiple components simultaneously. The consultations with people with FMD did not reveal the same difficulty when responding to such multi-unit questions.

Delays in responding to questions were another interactional feature that distinguished people with FMD from people with dementia. The latter typically either did not respond to questions, which prompted further questioning or clarification from the clinician, or their responses were delayed, sometimes substantially (e.g. on occasion almost 10 seconds before the patient produced a response) and therefore were treated as noticeable and accountable by both the neurologist and accompanying person, who often sought to repair the situation.

The final feature dealt with patients' abilities to provide detailed accounts in their answers to the clinician's questions. When comparing the responses of the different patient groupings it was evident that people with FMD were often able to provide both lengthy and detailed answers, comprising new and unsolicited information, which displayed the person's episodic memory capabilities. Responses by people with dementia, however, often consisted of admissions of forgetfulness or a lack of understanding, for example 'Can't remember now' (Jones et al., 2016, p. 505). In contrast to the elaborated accounts provided by people with FMD, the answers by people with dementia were also very short single-utterance or single-turn units that did not provide any additional or voluntary information. This is exemplified in Excerpt 3.

Excerpt 3 (DOC=Doctor, PAT=Patient, OTH=Companion)

```
01  DOC: .hh so we- we've discussed your memory at
02       wo:rk, how'd- ho:w do you feel your (.)
03       memory is: (.) at ho:me?
04       (0.2)
05  PAT: er: (0.2) not too good.
06       (0.3)
07  DOC: not too good.
08       (0.7) ((Neurologist writing))
09  DOC: .h could you: tell me a bit more about tha:t?
10       (.)
11  PAT: tch um:: (10.1)((Patient looks to companion))
12  OTH: you can't find things any more.
```

The neurologist is here closing the discussion about the patient's memory problems 'at work' and focusing on additional issues he may face at home, seeking examples of the patient's experiences (lines 01 and 02). After some delay the patient admits to his memory not being 'too good' (line 05). The patient here does not elaborate on his response or provide any examples of instances when his memory failed. This unsolicited elaboration is often evident in cases when the person has FMD. Instead the neurologist pursues some elaboration by asking the patient to tell him 'a bit more' about his memory-failure experiences (line 09). The patient is unable to produce any detailed description of his memory problems and, after a lengthy delay of 10 seconds, turns to his companion for help. It is the companion who produces the detail required. These features, of people either not being able to answer a question (and thus relying on others to articulate the response on their behalf) or producing undetailed minimal responses, are recurrent interactional practices contributing to the interactional profiles of people with dementia.

The excerpts above have demonstrated different interactional patterns that can be used to distinguish dementia from FMD. In Jones et al. (2016), all participants were native English speakers. In the next section, we will present examples from a situation in which the interaction between clinician and patient is mediated by an interpreter.

Interpreter-mediated dementia evaluations

As explicated above, the dementia evaluation is a complex procedure, in which many different steps are taken and different instruments are used. New diagnostic means are also developed, such as the one reported on in the prior section, and existing tests and instruments are continuously improved. A spe-cific challenge for memory clinics, however, is that many instruments, for example tests of cognitive functioning, are not adapted to people of all eth-nicities nor translated or validated in all languages needed and rarely take limited literacy skills into account (e.g. Nielsen, 2011; Plejert et al., 2015). In addition, if a patient speaks a foreign language, it is routine in most memory clinics to appoint an interpreter to mediate the interaction between clinician and patient during the assessment. Although the field of research on interpret-ing in medical settings is vast (e.g. Angelelli, 2004; Karliner et al., 2007; Kaufert & Putsch, 1997), there are very few studies on interpreting in settings involving people with dementia (but cf. Van de Mieroop et al., 2012) and even fewer on the specific environment of memory clinic encounters. However, in two case-studies of interpreter-mediated dementia evaluations, Plejert et al. (2015) and Majlesi and Plejert (2016) investigated the interplay between interlocutors in this particular setting. Whereas the first study (Plejert et al., 2015) highlighted particular challenges associated with the lack of cultural and linguistic adaptation of a test of cognitive functioning to the patient, and how this lack of adaptation played out in interaction, the second one (Majlesi & Plejert, 2016) investigated how the clinician and interpreter used various embodied resources (e.g. pointing towards a watch, drawing a circle in the air as an iconic gesture for the face of a clock, etc.) in collaborative ways that in various manners potentially affected the patient's understanding and perfor-mance of the task at hand. This section primarily discusses some key findings from the initial case-study (Plejert et al., 2015) but also highlights some further aspects of the data that formed the basis for that study. The data comprised video recordings and ethnographic interviews collected in a Swedish memory clinic in 2013.

The participants in Plejert et al. (2015) are an experienced occupational therapist, a professional interpreter and a patient, an 80-year-old Iraqi Kurdish woman. Her mother tongue is a variety of Kurdish called Feyli, but she also appears to know some Arabic and Turkish. She has limited reading and writ-ing skills and knows how to count only to a small extent. The interpreter is asked to translate between Swedish and Kurdish. The analysis primarily focuses on the administration of a test of cognitive functioning, the Montreal Cogni-tive Assessment (MoCA) (Nasreddine, 2003). The MoCA is a screening instru-ment that assesses short-term memory (immediate and delayed recall of five nouns); visuospatial abilities (clock-drawing and three-dimensional cube-copy); executive functions (adapted Trail Making B, phonemic fluency and verbal abstraction); attention, concentration and working memory (target detection, serial subtraction and digits forward and backward); language (confrontation naming, repetition of two syntactically complex sentences and phonetic fluency); and orientation in time and place. The test is available in many languages, but not Kurdish. The clinical staff in the memory clinic claimed that they experienced that the test most of the time worked reasonably well when mediated by an interpreter. In addition, and importantly, they were very cautious about basing their diagnosis on a combination of results from the overall assessment – the test of cognitive functioning was but one part out of many, and in case of any uncertainties, they would exclude results. However, as clinicians stated themselves, it was often somewhat problematic for them to make informed inferences from patients' performances when interaction was mediated by an interpreter. They felt, at times, uncertain about whether what they, or the patient, had said had been rendered appropriately. As one physician said in an interview, 'we get what the patients are saying, but the *nuances* are missing'.

The skills and proficiency of the interpreter are naturally crucial for the process of assessment. Despite the fact that very many interpreters are highly skilled, there is, in Sweden and elsewhere, a lack of certified interpreters with a medical specialization in all the required languages (and varieties). And even with an advanced knowledge of medical interpreting, some tasks may be particularly demanding, such as interpreting that involves people with cognitive decline, such as dementia, or psychiatric conditions (cf. Bot, 2003, 2005, on interpreting in mental health), where patients' contributions and responses may deviate from what is ordinarily expected. If the interpreter is not specifically trained to handle such contributions, it may be the case that the interpreter tries to make sense of what has been said or selects to render what he or she perceives as 'medically relevant' (Bolden, 2000).

It should be pointed out that very many interpreter-mediated dementia evaluations work very well. The following excerpt, however, demonstrates an example of the kind of challenges that all participants (not only the patient) are faced with, due to the fact that a test at hand is linguistically and culturally biased. Excerpts 4a–d below come from the language part of the MoCA; the patient is to repeat a syntactically complex sentence. In Swedish, the sentence reads: 'Jag vet att det är Johan som ska få hjälp idag,' and in English: 'I know that it is Johan who will get help today.' The complexity lies in the original sentence comprising two subordinate clauses; a that clause (that it is Johan) and a relative clause (who will get help today). However, in Kurdish, relative clauses are not as common and not always used in the same ways as in Germanic languages such as Swedish and English, and this potentially affects the interpreter's rendition (among other things). Right before Excerpt 4a starts, the occupational therapist (OT) has given the formal instructions, and these instructions have been rendered to the patient (PAT) in Kurdish by the interpreter (INT). The OT then produces the sentence to be repeated (line 01). A translation into idiomatic English is found in *italics* beneath each line of original language (Swedish, or Kurdish).

Excerpt 4a (OT=Occupational therapist, INT=Interpreter, PAT=Patient)

```
01  OT:   m↑ .t .hhh jag vet att det är johan som ska få
          hjälp idag
          m↑ .t .hhh I know that it is johan who will get
          help today
02        (0.4)
03  INT:  på svenska >°eller°<↑
          in swedish >°or°<↑
04        (0.3)
05  OT:   .t nej på::.t no in::
06        (0.8)
07  INT:  aizheh (0.6) aizheh m- (0.4) hhh .hhh aizheh me
          azanem (2.2) she says (0.6) she says (0.4) she
          says hhh hhh I know (2.2)
08        alan aizhema awa o khot aidi beka peshtem=
          I tell it now and you should repeat it after me
09  PAT:  a:
10        (0.3)
11  INT:  me azanem (0.3) johan masalan ye- komaki (0.6)
          akaiman I know (0.3) johan for example this-
          help him (0.6)we do
12        (0.3)
13  PAT:  a:
14        (1.0)
```

As can be observed, the interpreter is a bit confused whether the task is to be performed in Swedish or Kurdish (line 03), which may be due to the fact that the test material is in Swedish, so he must not only interpret, but also translate text at this point. Also, it is noticeable that after the nature of the task has been clarified, he once more repeats to the patient what the task is about (lines 07 and 08), which is acknowledged by the patient (line 09). The interpreter's first version of the sentence to be repeated is then produced (line 11) 'I know (0.3) Johan for example this-help him (0.6) we do.' The fact that the word order is different in Kurdish is to be expected, since the two languages differ significantly in this respect (Kurdish having a less regulated word order), but already at this point, the complexity of the sentence has been somewhat reduced. The interpreter has also omitted the temporal term 'today', which he notices, and then subsequently he provides a new sample sentence to be repeated. This is illustrated in Excerpt 4b:

Excerpt 4b

```
01   INT:  emro komak johan akaiman
           today help johan we do
02   PAT:  a
```

It can be noticed that in this second version (line 01), the syntactic complexity is entirely missing with no subordinate clauses. It should be added that throughout this task the patient has difficulty understanding what she is supposed to do. She continuously provides acknowledgement tokens as if she understands (e.g. line 02, Excerpt 4b, and line 13, Excerpt 4a) but does not repeat the test sentence until the interpreter finds out a way by asking the patient what he had just said (Excerpt 4c, line 03):

Excerpt 4c

```
01   PAT: bizhem cha
          what should I say
02        (0.5)
03   INT: cha wetem me(n)
          what did I say
04        (0.7)
05   PAT: veti komake miwan akain
          you said help guest we do
```

The patient eventually repeats the sentence (line 05). Her version is similar to the interpreter's (Excerpt 4b, line 01), apart from leaving out the temporal 'today' and exchanging the name Johan to the Kurdish word 'miwan', meaning 'guest'. It should be noticed that prosodically, 'Johan' (the way the interpreter pronounces it) and 'miwan' share the same stress-pattern. In addition, the pronunciation of the second syllables of both words is the same. The fact that, throughout the interaction, the patient displays hearing difficulties may also have had an impact on what might be considered a rather qualified 'guess' of a word that fits the overall meaning of the sentence.

The cultural bias of the task is also clearly visible here, since the name Johan does not exist in Kurdish. This fact might be an alternative explanation for the patient's attempt to find another word that fits the context. This leads to further repair-work between patient and interpreter, during which the patient attempts to provide a name that exists in Kurdish, namely 'Borhan':

Excerpt 4d

```
01   INT: =na mevan YOHAN
          =not guest JOHAN
02   PAT: borhan↑
03   INT: joh- hh he [he he]
04   PAT:           [(x x x]
05   INT: [de blir svårt me] namnet
          [it is difficult with] the name
06   OT:  [ja::::::]
          [yea:::::]
```

```
07        (0.8)
08   OT:  a de ä svårt o komma i[hågↂ  (0.2) tror jag
          faktiskt] så: eh a it is hard to re[member (0.2)
          I think actually] so: eh
```

The interpreter performs cultural brokerage (e.g. Kaufert & Koolage, 1984) and explains to the occupational therapist that the name Johan is difficult (line 05). However, at this point, and probably because the occupational therapist has not received sufficient renditions of the repair-work demonstrated in Excerpts 4a–c, she appears to interpret the patient's difficulties to perform the task as a memory difficulty (line 08).

Diagnostic disclosure

An important aspect of diagnostic pathways is the delivery of the diagnosis. As we discussed in the introduction, people may orient quite differently towards receiving a dementia diagnosis. Some are perhaps relieved and really want to know their diagnosis, whereas others might experience the diagnosis as stigmatising or inappropriate. Some research suggests, however, that 'catastrophic' reactions to a dementia diagnosis are fairly uncommon (e.g. Lecouturier et al., 2008). Historically, it was thought that people with dementia need not be well informed about the diagnosis or the disease. However, this attitude has now changed, and it is believed that a person with potential dementia 'has the right to know' (Bamford et al., 2004; Hellström & Torres, 2013, p. 158). Nonetheless, it is still the case that clinicians might tend to avoid explicitly using terminology such as 'dementia' or 'Alzheimer's disease' with the patient themselves (Karnieli-Miller et al., 2007; Peel, 2015). This is perhaps also reflected in the choice of the label 'memory clinic' for specialist services, rather than more explicit terms such as 'dementia service', although, in the United Kingdom, for example, there has been a move in some memory services to label them as more explicitly a dementia-related service, for instance the Worcestershire Early Intervention Dementia Service (La Fontaine et al., n.d.). In part, the use of the term dementia in the title of the service acts as a counter to the (potentially) obfuscatory and 'veiled' language often encountered in dementia health service provision (Karnieli-Miller et al., 2007). This degree of clarity about diagnostic service delivery is not, however, normative, and a fundamental issue is how diagnostic disclosure is communicated by clinicians, how it is received by patients and relatives and how diagnosis can 'best' be delivered.

The vast majority of research on dementia diagnostic disclosure is based on surveys, or in some cases interviews, primarily with clinicians (physicians, psychiatrists, neurologists, etc.) or relatives of people with dementia, and in a few cases also turning to people with dementia (e.g. Clare, 2003) or people waiting to see a physician (Erde et al., 1998). A systematic review on dementia disclosure by Bamford et al. (2004) presented a highly intricate and complex picture of this field of research, outlining seven major themes: (1) whether people with dementia should be told their diagnosis, (2) aspects of the process of disclosing and receiving a diagnosis of dementia, (3) studies of reported practice, (4) reasons for and against disclosure, (5) factors influencing disclosure, (6) impacts of disclosure, and (7) carers' experience of disclosure. From their review, Bamford et al. (2004, pp. 165–166) concluded that 'for many practitioners, patients and carers, disclosing a diagnosis of dementia is neither inevitable nor straightforward', and they suggested that 'qualitative research is needed to increase our understanding of the process of disclosure and enable people with dementia and their carers to obtain as much, or as little, information about their diagnosis as they want' (ibid., p. 167). While the question of *whether* people with a probable dementia should be told their diagnosis has largely receded from the academic literature and current Western health-care practice, there is great nuance and variability in how the diagnostic process proceeds, bearing in mind variations in individuals' cognitive and communicative abilities, degree of insight and (potential) co-morbidities. Recent research using focus groups and interviews with current medical students, for example, highlights that deception remains a live issue in the context of dementia health care and that issues of capacity, perceived vulnerability and family dynamics all complicate clinical judgments in the dementia care context (Tullo et al., 2015), and this likely impacts on clinical communication.

A recent study that provides exactly the kind of empirical evidence called for by Bamford et al. (2004) is a CA study by Peel (2015) on diagnostic communication in a memory clinic. As mentioned, CA methodology facilitates analyses of participants' moment-by-moment interactional practices and orientations. In interactions involving clinicians and patients with dementia and their relatives, it is therefore possible to closely study specific conversational actions, and how such actions are immediately responded and reacted to, for instance the comparison between responses to questions by people with FMDs and people with dementia that we discussed above. Concerning questions such as, for example, whether a person with dementia should or should not be told their diagnosis, or, if clinicians avoid terms such as 'dementia' and 'Alzheimer's disease', by means of CA it is possible to observe how these features are played out during real-time interaction. This is an important complement to results from survey and interview studies (particularly also since self-reports might not always reflect people's actual practices). The literature on clinicians' self-reports of their diagnostic disclosure practices, for example, demonstrates that they are able to articulate their practices, such as putting a 'positive spin' on the diagnosis (Kissel & Carpenter, 2007, p. 277), but this does not offer a lens through which to scrutinise the process itself. Nor does this type of research illuminate how their professed approach to diagnostic delivery is received by patients and relatives. Let us now turn to excerpts from Peel (2015) that demonstrate the actual process of diagnostic disclosure in a UK memory clinic. The data-set as a whole comprised video-recordings of 29 patients and accompanying persons attending a rural memory service, all of whom were white and native English speakers. Overall there were six interactions during which the old-age psychiatrist was evaluating the patient's condition (Heritage & Maynard, 2006). In Excerpts 5a and 5b below it is the patient's daughter (DAU) who seeks clarification about her mother's (PAT) brain scan.

Excerpt 5a (DR: Doctor, DAU: Daughter) (taken from Peel, 2015, p. 1125)

```
01   DAU: so w-was the- the sca:n that was all oka::y (.)
02        >I think< wasn't it.
03   DR.: the- the- the scan shows w-well i-it .hh so:me-
          er some changes
04        that- that- that occur as we get older=
05   DAU: °mhm°
06   DR.: =that is there are- there's no tu:mours, there's
          no vascular, no
07        BI:g vessel changes=
08   DAU: mhm.
09   DR.: =that are demonstrated but- but there- there is
          a degree of
10        redu:ced er volume
11   DAU: mhm.
12   DR.: of er brain substance .hh and that's significant ...
```

Here the daughter starts to ask a question ('so was the—') which she then self-repairs to a declarative question about the outcome of her mother's brain scan. When the doctor does not start his turn at 'okay' she downgrades her epistemic authority (Heritage & Raymond, 2005) in deference to the doctor ('I think'). Through her reformulated question the daughter is seeking clarification on the outcome from the scan in a way that positions a problem as a dispreferred next turn ('all okay') but also places the clinician in position of high epistemic authority. The diagnosis conveyed in lines 03a–04, 06–07, 09–10 and 12 starts with 'well', which projects that the answer is not going to be straightforward (Schegloff & Lerner, 2009) and initially normalises the scan results ('some changes that occur as we get older') and reports on what the scan did not find, before mentioning the 'significance' of reduced brain volume, which is typical in Alzheimer's disease. We turn now to the close of this interaction.

Excerpt 5b (DR=Doctor, DAU: Daughter, PAT=Patient)

```
01   DAU: yep.
02   DR.: okay.
03   DAU: mhmm.
04   PAT: oh well t'hh thank you very much for your ti::me.
```

We can see in Excerpts 5a and 5b that, contrary to Karnieli-Miller et al.'s (2012) observation that by the end of the diagnostic encounter the person with dementia is being ignored, something more complex is occurring. The doctor's shift in focus to the patient's daughter, rather than the patient herself, has been *prompted* by the daughter, and the patient herself draws the exchange to a close. At this point the video shows the patient holding her head before moving her hand away as she says 'oh well' in line 04, suggesting both a tacit acknowledgement of the information and (perhaps) an acceptance of its inevitability. But 'thank you very much for your time' arguably steps away from a more explicit articulation of receipt of this information (a thanking for information or expertise) through this more formulaic closing. These examples show perhaps a normative degree of patient acknowledgement of diagnostic information, delivered with sensitivity to the concerns of the caring dyad rather than simply the patient as an individual. By contrast, the final example is taken from a consultation in which the term 'Alzheimer's' is explicitly and unambiguously used by the clinician.

Excerpt 6: (DR=Doctor, PAT=Patient) (taken from Peel, 2015, p. 1127)

```
01   DR.: well it [brain scan] showed some: changes and
           on that basis and
02         your [clinical condition
03   PAT:      [W-
04   DR:  we do say that you have the early stages of
           Alzheimer cha:nges
05         that's why you're on the treatment that you're on.

[32 lines omitted]

06   PAT: er but I was also told by another grocer who'd
           had a breakdown
07         he said "your memory wi:ll come back" and I
           didn't rea:lly (.)
08         believe him but it is coming (.) back.
```

What this excerpt clearly highlights is that there is – at least for this patient at this time – no necessary correspondence between the explicit use of the term Alzheimer's and a recognition and understanding that a dementia is what he is experiencing. Therefore CA-informed analysis can bring into question the current assumption that the use of explicit terminology (e.g. Alzheimer's) is inherently important to the appropriate communication of diagnosis.

Concluding discussion

The aim of this chapter was to foreground different components of the dementia diagnosis pathways. By way of discussion, we will explore more precisely the clinical and practical implications generated by the studies reported on above.

Beginning with the study by Jones et al. (2016), we showed how results from detailed analyses of interlocutors' interactional contributions may assist in diagnosing memory problems and differentiating dementia from non-organic FMD. These findings, and the resulting profiles, could underpin an interactional toolkit to aid practitioners in designing their consultation to maximise diagnostic potential and provide concrete grounds to support clinicians' intuitive formations of a 'working diagnosis' during the first couple of minutes of an initial consultation. It should be pointed out, however, that the study reports initial observations that need to be developed further to become an additional diagnostic method in memory clinics. To date, these candidate diagnostic interactional features have been developed into a working diagnostic scoring tool and blind tested by two linguistic coders against ten patients (five with confirmed FMD diagnosis and five with dementia) to check inter-rater reliability and the diagnostic accuracy of the distinctive conversational profiles (Elsey et al., 2015). The results appear promising, particularly in terms of enabling a more speedy diagnosis, and for potentially sparing patients extensive and burdensome neuropsychological testing. Additionally, the toolkit could be used in other services within the diagnostic pathway, including general practitioners in primary care who are increasingly required to 'screen' for dementia. It may help to ensure patients are being referred to appropriate secondary services (e.g. counselling services for patients with functional memory complaints resulting from anxiety or depression) and reduce the burden on memory clinic services. Using conversation as a method of assessment throughout the assessment pathway could therefore be of significant diagnostic value.

When it comes to the study of the interpreter-mediated dementia assessments, it demonstrates the many interactional details that may influence not just the actual administration of different parts of cognitive evaluation, but also how, for example, patients' performances on different parts of a test are to be assessed. In Excerpts 4a–d, the interpreter and the patient got involved in a series of repair-sequences concerning the patient's lack of understanding of the task, her potential hearing difficulty and the fact that the name to be repeated was (culturally) unfamiliar to her. In addition, the interpreter appeared strongly oriented towards making the patient carry out the task in the way asked for by the occupational therapist. This potentially contributed to his not consistently rendering what was being said during the repair. Analysis of the transcript, however, revealed that several interactional actions were of potentially great relevance from a diagnostic point of view, details unavailable for the clinician. Also, despite the fact that the interpreter did attempt to explain that the culturally unfamiliar name was probably contributing to the patient's difficulties, the lack of access to what had been going on during repair eventually influenced the occupational therapist's interpretation of the patient's performance of the task.

These findings suggest that optimally, interpreter-mediated encounters should be recorded, transcribed and translated and the transcriptions subsequently screened by the clinicians involved in the evaluation. However, such a process would be much too costly and time-consuming, and also ethically problematic, since all patients would perhaps not give their consent to being audio recorded or video recorded. The findings also support current developments of tests that are more adapted to patients with limited reading and writing skills, and less culture dependent, for example the Rowland Universal Assessment Scale (RUDAS) (see Naqvi et al., 2015). To use such tests probably also facilitates the interpreter's task. This, however, remains to be investigated further, preferably using CA. Finally, our observations also signal that further interpreter training is needed, particularly concerning formal medical tasks, such as neuropsychological tests. In relation to the current steep increase in Sweden, and worldwide, in immigrant populations, there are discussions (in Sweden) at the national level concerning developing special 'short-cuts' in interpreter training. This is worrying, considering the challenges already facing interpreters in terms of often not having enough training for mediating talk during quite specific clinical tasks or encounters involving people with potential cognitive impairments. If anything, more training is needed, rather than less, to secure assessment accuracy.

When it comes to dementia disclosure, we demonstrated in Excerpts 5a and 5b how the diagnosis may be communicated in a 'veiled' way (Bergmann, 1992), as the seriousness of the diagnosis is communicated through the words 'significant' and 'changes' rather than through the direct use of terms like Alzheimer's disease. Overall, this example would suggest that while explicit diagnostic information (i.e. probable Alzheimer's disease) is not delivered, the receipt of the information is in step with diagnostic delivery (i.e. minimal) as it occurs in other medical settings and conforms to the intersubjective norms of minimizing catastrophic reactions in medical communication (Maynard & Frankel, 2006). Rather than dementia diagnosis delivery necessarily being a 'special case', in keeping with the receipt of diagnostic information in other medical contexts (e.g. Heath, 1992) this information is not received as news but is minimally received by the daughter and met with silence from the patient. Nevertheless, these interactions highlight not only the considerable complexity at work within this context but also knotty interpersonal and family dynamics, which are being managed on an unfolding basis (Peel, 2015; Riggs & Peel,

2016). By contrast, Excerpt 6 demonstrated that the use of explicit diagnostic terms does not necessarily improve patients' understanding or awareness of their condition. Therefore, CA analyses may enable us to trouble the notion in the existing literature (e.g. Karnieli-Miller et al., 2007) that health professionals' not typically using the words Alzheimer's or dementia in interactions with patients is fundamentally problematic and obfuscatory and to further a more nuanced understanding of the interactional processes involved in communicating diagnosis. How these interactional processes map onto different 'types' of patients and caring dyads or triads, in terms of being mediated by culture–ethnicity, gender, social class, age and level of (dis)ability, is yet to be charted. But as the above examples across the three key aspects of dementia diagnostic practice (initial assessment, cognitive testing and diagnostic delivery) attest, CA offers a rich analytic seam through which to mine, and ultimately inform, diagnostic pathways and practices in dementia care.

As our discussion of these three aspects within the dementia diagnosis pathway has highlighted, a close focus on how, and in what ways, interactions unfold can illuminate a range of components in dementia care. By closely exploring dementia care as it is actually enacted (rather than relying on second-hand reports) there is the potential to understand how the diagnostic experience can be improved for health professionals, family carers and, most importantly, people living with dementia themselves. Understanding how diagnostic interactions work in practice can potentially assist in improving practice. Ultimately, improved practice impacts on better patient experience, which may contribute to better adjustment to living with dementia in the long term.

Transcription conventions (adapted from Jefferson, 2004)

=	Links talk produced in close temporal proximity (latched talk)
><	Talk between symbols is rushed or compressed
°°	Encloses talk which is produced quietly
underline	Underlining marks emphasis of some kind
CAPS	Words or parts of words spoken loudly marked in capital letters
s:::::	Sustained or stretched sound; the more colons, the longer the sound
. ?,	Stop indicates falling intonation; a question mark indicates rising intonation over a word; a comma indicates a slight rising intonation at the end of a word

.hhh	Inbreath, the number of 'h's representing the length of the inbreath
hhh.	Outbreath, the number of 'h's representing the length of the outbreath
[]	Encloses talk in overlap i.e. when more than one speaker is speaking
(word)	Parentheses indicate transcriber doubt
(this/that)	Alternative hearings
((description))	Description of what can be heard, rather than transcription e.g.
((shuffling	papers))
cu-	Cut-off word or sound
(0.6)	Silence in seconds
(.)	Silence of less than two-tenths of a second
∧ or ↑	Indicates marked pitch rise
∨ or ↓	Indicates marked fall in pitch
(hhenhh)	Indicates laughter while speaking (aspiration)

Acknowledgements

The research on which this chapter is based was funded by Riksbankens Jubile-umsfond – The Swedish Foundation for Humanities and Social Sciences (grant number M10-0187:1), the National Institute for Health Research (NIHR) under its Research for Patient Benefit (RfPB) Programme (grant number PB-PG-0211-24079) and a British Academy Mid-Career Fellowship (grant number MC110142).

References

Adelman, A. M. & Daly, M. P. (2005). Initial evaluation of the patient with suspected dementia. *American Family Physician, 71*, 1745–1750.

Angelelli, C. V. (2004). *Medical Interpreting and Cross-Cultural Communication*. Cambridge: Cambridge University Press.

Antaki, C. (2011). *Applied Conversation Analysis*. Basingstoke: Palgrave-Macmillan.

Bamford, C., Lamont, S., Eccles, M., Robinson, L., May, C. & Bond, J. (2004). Disclosing a diagnosis of dementia: A systematic review. *International Journal of Geriatric Psychiatry, 19*, 151–169.

Bergmann, J. R. (1992). Veiled morality: Notes on discretion in psychiatry. In P. Drew & J. Heritage (Eds.), *Talk at Work* (pp. 137–162). Cambridge: Cambridge University Press.

Blackburn, D. J., Wakefield, S., Shanks, M. F., Harkness, K., Reuber, M. & Venneri, A. (2014). Memory difficulties are not always a sign of incipient dementia: A review of the possible causes of loss of memory efficiency. *British Medical Bulletin, 112,* 71–81.

Bolden, B. G. (2000). Towards understanding practices of medical interpreting: Interpreters' involvement in history taking. *Discourse Studies, 2,* 387–419.

Bot, H. (2003). The myth of the uninvolved interpreter in mental health and the development of a three-person psychology. In. L. Brunette, G. Bastin, I. Hemlin & H. Clarke (Eds.), *The Critical Link3* (pp. 27–35). Amsterdam & Philadelphia: John Benjamins.

Bot, H. (2005). *Dialogue Interpreting in Mental Health.* Amsterdam & New York: Rodopi Publishers.

Brooker, D., La Fontaine, J., Evans, S., Bray, J. & Saad, K. (2014). Public health guidance to facilitate timely diagnosis of dementia: Alzheimer's Cooperative Valuation in Europe recommendations. *International Journal of Geriatric Psychiatry, 29,* 682–693.

Chatwin, J. (2014). Conversation analysis as a method for investigating interaction in care home environments. *Dementia, 13,* 737–746.

Clare, L. (2003). Managing threats to self: Awareness in early stage Alzheimer's disease. *Social Science & Medicine, 57,* 1017–1029.

Dilworth-Anderson, P. & Gibson, B. (2002). The cultural influence of values, norms, meanings, and perceptions in understanding dementia in ethnic minorities. *Alzheimer Disease and Associated Disorders, 16,* 56–63.

Dilworth-Anderson, P., Williams, I. C. & Gibson, B. F. (2002). Issues of race, ethnicity, and culture in caregiving research: A 20-year review (1980–2000). *The Gerontologist, 42,* 237–272.

Drew, P. (2005). Conversation analysis. In K. L. Fitch & R. E. Sanders (Eds.), *Handbook of Language and Social Interaction* (pp. 71–102). London: Lawrence Erlbaum Associates Publishers.

Elsey, C., Drew, P., Jones, D., Blackburn, D., Wakefield, S., Harkness, K., Venneri, A. & Reuber, M. (2015). Towards diagnostic conversational profiles of patients presenting with dementia or functional memory disorders to memory clinics. *Patient Education and Counseling, 98,* 1071–1077.

Erde, E. L., Nadal, E. C. & Scholl, T. O. (1988). On truth telling and the diagnosis of Alzheimer's disease. *Journal of Family Practice, 26,* 401–406.

Erol, R., Brooker, D. & Peel, E. (2015). *Women and Dementia: A Global Research Review.* London: Alzheimer's Disease International. Available at www.alz.co.uk/women-and-dementia, accessed 10 February 2017.

Goodwin. C. (2003). *Conversation and Brain Damage.* Oxford: Oxford University Press.

Heath, C. (1992). The delivery and reception of diagnosis and assessment in the general practice consultation. In P. Drew & J. Heritage (Eds.), *Talk at Work* (pp. 235–267). Cambridge: Cambridge University Press.

Hellström, I. & Torres, S. (2013). A wish to know but not always tell – Couples living with dementia talk about disclosure preferences. *Aging & Mental Health, 17,* 157–167.

Heritage, J. & Maynard, D. W. (2006). Introduction: Analyzing interaction between doctors and patients in primary care encounters. In J. Heritage & D. W. Maynard (Eds.), *Communication in Medical Care* (pp. 1–21). New York: Cambridge University Press.

Heritage, J. & Raymond, G. (2005). The terms of agreement: Indexing epistemic authority and subordination in talk-in-interaction. *Social Psychology Quarterly, 68*, 15–38.

Heritage, J., Robinson, J., Elliott, M., Beckett, M. & Wilkes, M. (2007). Reducing patients' unmet concerns in primary care: The difference one word can make. *Journal of General Internal Medicine, 22*, 1429–1433.

Hydén, L. C., Samuelsson, C., Örulv, L. & Plejert, C. (2012). Feedback in narrative interaction involving people with dementia. *Journal of Interactional Research in Communication Disorders, 4*, 211–247.

Jefferson, G. (2004). Glossary of transcript symbols with an introduction. In G. H. Lerner (Ed.), *Conversation Analysis: Studies from the First Generation* (pp. 13–23). Philadelphia, PA: John Benjamins.

Jones, D. (2015). A family living with Alzheimer's disease: The communicative challenges. *Dementia: The International Journal of Social Research and Practice, 14*(5), 555–573.

Jones, D., Drew, P., Elsey, C., Blackburn, D., Wakefield, S., Harkness, K. & Reuber, M. (2016). Conversational assessment in memory clinic encounters: Interactional profiling for differentiating dementia from functional memory disorders. *Aging & Mental Health, 20*, 500–509.

Karliner, L. S., Jacobs, E. A., Hm Chen, A. & Mutha, S. (2007). Do professional interpreters improve clinical care for patients with limited English proficiency? A systematic review of the literature. *Health Services Research, 42*, 727–748.

Karnieli-Miller, O., Werner, P., Aharon-Peretz, J. & Eidelman, S. (2007). Dilemmas in the (un)veiling of the diagnosis of Alzheimer's disease: Walking an ethical and professional tight rope. *Patient Education and Counseling, 67*, 307–314.

Karnieli-Miller, O., Werner, P., Neufeld-Kroszynski, G. & Eidelman, S. (2012). Are you talking to me?! An exploration of the triadic physician–patient–companion communication within memory clinics encounters. *Patient Education and Counseling, 88*, 381–390.

Kaufert, J. & Putsch, R. (1997). Communication through interpreters in healthcare: Ethical dilemmas arising from differences in class, culture, language and power. *The Journal of Clinical Ethics, 8*, 71–87.

Kaufert, J. M. & Koolage, W. W. (1984). Role conflict among 'culture brokers': The experience of native Canadian medical interpreters. *Social Science and Medicine, 18*, 283–286.

Kissel, E. C. & Carpenter, B. D. (2007). It's all in the details: Physician variability in disclosing a dementia diagnosis. *Aging & Mental Health, 3*, 273–280.

LaFontaine, J., Brooker, D., Wallcraft, J. & Vickers, H. (n.d.). Evaluation Report Early Intervention Dementia Service Worcestershire. University of Worcester: Association for Dementia Studies.

Lecouturier, J., Bamford, C., Hughes, J. C., Francis, J. J., Foy, R. & Eccles, P. M. (2008). Appropriate disclosure of a diagnosis of dementia: Identifying the key behaviours of 'best practice'. *BMC Health Services Research, 8*, 95. doi:10.1186/1472-6963-8-95.

Leibing, A. & Cohen, L. (2006). *Thinking about Dementia: Culture, Loss, and the Anthropology of Senility.* New Brunswick, NJ: Rutgers University Press.

Linell, P., Hofvendahl, J. & Lindholm, C. (2003). Multi-unit questions in institutional interactions: Sequential organizations and communicative functions. *Text, 23*, 539–571.

Majlesi, A. R. & Plejert, C. (2016). Embodiment in tests of cognitive functioning: A study of an interpreter-mediated dementia evaluation. *Dementia.* Published online first 27 February 2016. doi:101177/1471301216635341.

Maynard, D. W. & Frankel, R. M. (2006). On diagnostic rationality: Bad news, good news, and the symptom residue. In J. Heritage & D. W. Maynard (Eds.), *Communication in Medical Care* (pp. 248–278). New York: Cambridge University Press.

Nasreddine, Z. (2003–2014). The Montreal Cognitive Assessment MoCA©.

Naqvi, M. R., Halder, S., Tomlinson, G. & Alibhai, S. (2015). Cognitive assessments in multicultural populations using the Rowland Universal Dementia Assessment Scale: A systematic review and meta-analysis. *Canadian Medical Association Journal, 187*(5), E169–E175.

Nielsen, T. R. (2011). *Evaluation of dementia in patients from ethnic minorities. A European perspective.* PhD dissertation, Copenhagen University.

O'Connor, D. W., Pollitt, P. A. & Treasure, F. P. (1991). The influence of education and social class on the diagnosis of dementia in a community population. *Psychological Medicine, 21,* 219–224.

Peel, E. (2014). 'The living death of Alzheimer's' versus 'Take a walk to keep dementia at bay': Representations of dementia in print media and carer discourse. *Sociology of Health and Illness, 36,* 885–901.

Peel, E. (2015). Diagnostic communication in the memory clinic: A conversation analytic perspective. *Aging & Mental Health, 19,* 1123–1130.

Peel, E. & Harding, R. (2014). 'It's a huge maze, the system, it's a terrible maze': Dementia carers' constructions of navigating health and social care services. *Dementia: The International Journal of Social Research and Practice, 13,* 642–666.

Peel, E. & McDaid, S. (2015). *'Over the Rainbow': Lesbian, Gay, Bisexual, Trans People and Dementia Project. Summary Report.* University of Worcester. Available at: http://dementiavoices.org.uk/wp-content/uploads/2015/03/Over-the-Rainbow-LGBTDementia-Report.pdf, accessed 10 February 2017.

Plejert, C., Antelius, E., Yazdanpanah, M. & Nielsen, T. R. (2015). There's a letter called ef. On challenges and repair in interpreter-mediated tests of cognitive functioning in dementia evaluations: A case study. *Journal of Cross-Cultural Gerontology, 30,* 163–187.

Plug, L., Sharrack, B. & Reuber. M. (2011). Metaphors in the description of seizure experiences: Common conceptualisations and differential diagnosis. *Language and Cognition, 3,* 209–233.

Reuber, M., Monzoni, C., Sharrack, B. & Plug, L. (2009). Using conversation analysis to distinguish between epileptic and psychogenic non-epileptic seizures: A prospective blinded multi-rater study. *Epilepsy and Behavior, 16,* 139–144.

Riggs, D. W. & Peel, E. (2016). *Critical Kinship Studies: An Introduction to the Field.* London: Palgrave Macmillan.

Robson, C., Drew, P., Walker, T., & Reuber, M. (2012). Catastrophising and normalising in patient's accounts of their seizure experiences. *Seizure, 21,* 795–801.

Rosser, M. N., Fox, N. C., Mummery, C. J., Schott, J. M. & Warren, J. D. (2010). The diagnosis of young-onset dementia. *Lancet Neurology, 9,* 973–806.

Royal College of Psychiatrists (2013). English National Memory Clinic Audit Report. Retrieved from www.rcpsych.ac.uk/pdf/English%20National%20Memory%20Clinics%20Audit%20Report%202013.pdf, accessed 10 February 2017.

Sacks, H., Schegloff, E. A. & Jefferson, G. (1974). A simplest systematics for the organization of turn-taking for conversation. *Language, 50, 696–735.*

Samsi, K., Abley, C., Campbell, S., Keady, J., Manthorpe, J., Robinson, L., Watts, S. &
Bond, J. (2014). Negotiating a labyrinth: Experiences of assessment and diagnostic
journey in cognitive impairment and dementia. *International Journal of Geriatric
Psychiatry, 29, 58–67.*

Schegloff, E. A. (1996). Confirming allusions: Toward an empirical account of action.
American Journal of Sociology, 104, 161–216.

Schegloff, E. A. (2007). *Sequence Organization in Interaction: A Primer in Conversation
Analysis.* Cambridge : Cambridge University Press.

Schegloff, E. A., Jefferson, G. & Sacks, H. (1977). The preference for self-correction in the
organization of repair in conversation. *Language, 53, 361–382.*

Schegloff, E. A. & Lerner, G. H. (2009). Beginning to respond: Well-prefaced responses to
wh-questions. *Research on Language and Social Interaction, 42, 91–115.*

Schrauf, R. W. & Iris, M. (2011). Very long pathways to diagnosis among African
Americans and Hispanics with memory and behavioral problems associated with
dementia. *Dementia, 11, 743–763.*

Shadlen, M.-F., Larson, E. B., Gibbons, L., McCormick, W. C. & Teri, L. (1999). Alzheimer's disease symptom severity in Blacks and Whites. *American Geriatrics Society, 47,*
482–486.

Sidnell, J. & Stivers, T. (2013). *The Handbook of Conversation Analysis.* Chichester:
Wiley-Blackwell.

Stivers, T. (2007). *Prescribing under Pressure: Parent–Physician Conversations and
Antibiotics.* Oxford: Oxford University Press.

Tullo, E. S., Lee, R. P., Robinson, L. & Allan, L. (2015). Why is dementia different? Medical
students' views about deceiving people with dementia. *Aging and Mental Health, 19,*
731–738.

Van de Mieroop, D., Bevilacqua, G. & Van Hove, L. (2012). Negotiating discursive norms.
Community interpreting in a Belgian rest home. *Interpreting, 14, 23–54.*

6

COMMUNICATION AND COLLABORATION IN DEMENTIA

Anna Ekström, Camilla Lindholm, Ali Reza Majlesi and Christina Samuelsson

Introduction

Communication is one of the areas in which people with dementia and their conversational partners (including family caregivers or formal staff in care homes) experience the most challenges (Murphy et al., 2010; Saunders et al., 2012). It has repeatedly been shown that the ability to initiate and maintain interactions with other people declines as dementia progresses (e.g. Evans et al., 2007; Örulv & Nikku, 2007). As the ability to communicate is crucial for creating and maintaining social relations, a dementia disease increases the risk of social exclusion (Kitwood, 1997; Örulv & Hydén, 2006; Sabat, 2002). In interview studies, people living with dementia often describe the difficulties they have both initiating and maintaining social interactions and how they experience diminished social relationships (Ericsson et al., 2011; Saunders et al., 2012). This, in turn, may also contribute to a decreased quality of life for people with dementia (Saunders et al., 2012). Moreover, deteriorating communication not only affects a person's social relations but also increases stress and is associated with higher risk of mortality for people with dementia (Dunn et al., 1994; Schulz & O'Brien, 1994; Williamson & Schulz, 1993; Wright, 1993). As a person's communicative abilities decline, it becomes increasingly difficult to guarantee that the person's views are heard (Murphy et al., 2010).

However, even if some competences in cognitive and communicative domains become limited over time, people with dementia do not lose their entire functional capacity, and some cognitive and communicative domains may remain intact across the spectrum of dementia (see e.g. Clare, 2008). The commonly portrayed picture of people with dementia as uninvolved communicative partners is, in our perspective, both misleading and unfortunate. At times, communication with people with dementia may be characterized as atypical, but being observant in the ways of communication, people with dementia may also prove to be competent collaborative partners in various activities. In fact, collaboration in communication would pave the way for people with dementia to use their current competencies to communicate with others and to remain active in interactional situations.

In this chapter, we make use of two separate but interrelated approaches to describe and understand communication involving people with dementia: a dialogic perspective (Linell, 2009) and an emergent pragmatic approach (Perkins, 2007). Using these perspectives, we uphold that human communication is an inherently collaborative activity and constructed through the mutual engagement and cooperation of the interacting participants. By using examples of communication in everyday and institutional activities, we argue for the significance of an integrated approach to the use of verbal and nonverbal communicative resources (talk, gesture, tools, artefacts, etc.) in communication with people with dementia. The chapter details how collaboration may provide grounds for mutual understanding in communication, leading toward increasing engagement of people with dementia in actively cooperating and sharing responsibilities in interaction to accomplish different communicative activities.

Dementia and communication

Of all of the domains affected by dementia diseases, communication has been argued to be the most substantially impacted area (Alm et al., 2004; Azuma & Bayles, 1997). In dementia, communicative ability gradually deteriorates over time, typically causing a dramatic diminishment of communicative skills in the late stage. A significant characteristic of communication in dementia is semantic impairment (Guendouzi & Müller, 2006), while both syntactic and phonological processes usually remain fairly intact, at least in an early to mid stage of the disease (Perkins et al., 1998). In initial stages of dementia, specific linguistic symptoms, such as word-finding difficulties, may occur, but as the disease progresses the communicative problems increase, and the person with dementia may encounter difficulties in participating in conversations. Further, language comprehension may also be impaired (e.g. Bayles & Tomoeda, 2007). Communication might also be complicated by additional impairment in nonverbal skills in the later stages of the disease, for example by the decreased use of gesture and poor eye contact (Maxim & Bryan, 2006, p. 79).

Communication in dementia is often characterized by deficiency in both language processing and other cognitive functions supporting communication. Impaired executive functions may cause repetitive and stereotyped language (i.e. tendency to have ritualized behaviour or to repeat sentences, stories, jokes and gestures), which has been shown to be common for people with dementia (Bayles et al., 1985; Perkins, 2007). Working memory problems have also been demonstrated to be the source of referential deficits (e.g. in the form of excessive pronoun usage), rather than a problem with lexical semantics (Almor et al., 1999). All in all, it seems that a combination of problems with memory and executive functions underlies the poor word recall in dementia, particularly in Alzheimer's disease (AD) (Azuma & Bayles, 1997).

Hydén (in press) puts forward a number of problems related to communication and dementia identified from studies of both conversations and storytelling. As described by Hydén, people with dementia:

- with a beginning in the early stage of dementia, have difficulties finding words, use unexpected and seemingly irrelevant words or neologisms or pronounce words in an unusual way;

- have increasing difficulties to identify references to past events, persons or places;

- have difficulties managing discourse topics and will as a result make sudden topical shifts without advance warning to the listener about the upcoming shift or giving an account for introducing a new topic;

- often repeat things already said or re-describe events or stories already reported.

It is, however, important to remember that deficiencies will vary between individuals, and different problems interact with each other and form a specific communicative profile for each individual diagnosed with dementia. As pointed out by Perkins et al. (1998), even though particular combinations of problems have been associated with different forms of dementia, 'there is a vast amount of individual variability within diagnostic categories that is potentially obscured by presentation of group data' (p. 36).

Pragmatic problems, that is, problems in social interaction, are central features in dementia. Much of the previous research on pragmatic practices in dementia has primarily been carried out through analysis of the ability of the person with dementia to produce different forms of discourse, for example storytelling, picture description and clinical interviews (Hydén, in press; Perkins et al., 1998). As pointed out by Perkins et al. (1998), while these kinds of studies have provided important information regarding aspects such as communicative coherence, length of communication unit, rate of speech and numbers of information units or propositional forms, it has also been claimed that conversations during interviews or in test situations differ significantly from interactions that take place between people with dementia and their caregivers on a daily basis (Perkins et al., 1998; Ripich & Terrell, 1988). Studies based on data generated from task-oriented conversations have also been criticised for not taking into account the role of the conversational partner or contextual factors of the environment where the conversation takes place.

There is a growing body of studies in which it is argued that discursive abilities are better understood in terms of interactional achievements of the conversing partners together, rather than individual measurements of the communicative
deficits of the person with dementia (see e.g. Hamilton, 1994; Ramanathan,
1997; Perkins et al., 1998; Hydén, in press; cf. Goodwin, 2003). A closer look at
unfolding interactions with people with dementia will provide a more comprehensive picture, not just of the loss in the cognitive abilities of people with
dementia, but also of their competence and abilities to use their available
resources to communicate with others. A common difficulty ascribed to individuals with dementia is problems related to turn-taking in conversation: people
with dementia are believed to gradually lose the ability to produce conversational turns at appropriate places (see Sacks et al., 1974 for a discussion of the
turn-taking system in conversation). Hamilton (1994), however, suggests that
the turn-taking mechanism is an aspect that remains relatively intact as the
disease progresses. Also in later stages of dementia, people are able to produce
their turns at the right place in conversation. Nonetheless, given the precise
timing required when producing a turn in conversation, cognitive deficiencies
may make it difficult for a person with dementia to take control over the conversational floor and to hold on to it for a long period of time (Perkins et al.,
1998). This is especially true in multiparty conversations in which the person
with dementia may just not be able to produce a turn quickly enough to secure
the position as a next speaker (cf. Causino Lamar et al., 1995; Sabat, 1991).
As described by Hydén (in press), for a person with dementia, partaking in a
multiparty conversation is demanding in several ways; following an ongoing
conversation, coming up with a possible contribution and identifying a potential time for delivering this contribution in a way that maintains the conversational flow can be challenging. A consequence of this might be that the person
with dementia would only be able to contribute to the conversation when
explicitly given the floor by another speaker. Moreover, people with dementia
may produce long pauses in their own conversational turns, which may lead to
a conversational partner taking over the floor. The complex demands of this
kind of communicative activity could lead to a situation in which the person
with dementia completely withdraws from the activity (Hydén, in press).

Communication and dementia from a dialogic and an emergentist approach to communication and dementia

The linguistic and communicative problems that have been demonstrated in
dementia have contributed to a view of people with dementia as incompetent
interactional partners whose language is incoherent or even meaningless. Such

views may make people enter conversation with a preconception that little of what the person with dementia says is comprehensible (Sabat, 1994). Communicative ability, however, means more than just an ability to transfer information; it is the site for human interaction, and primordially, a site for human sociality (Schegloff, 1987, p. 101). Put differently, communicative ability is a means for people to create and maintain human intersubjective relations, which also contributes to people's upholding of their personhood, identity and quality of life (see Hydén et al., 2014). Communication is by nature a collaborative activity, which requires contributions of co-interactants (Sacks et al., 1974). Thus, to what extent a person with dementia is able to participate in conversation depends not only on the severity of the communicative problems he or she encounters but also on the actions of interlocutors (Hamilton, 1994; Perkins et al., 1998; Ramanathan-Abbot, 1994; Sabat, 1994). In order to create a communicative situation that is beneficial for people with dementia, it is important to focus on well-functioning communicative strategies rather than on specific linguistic or communicative problems. It is also critical to highlight types of responses from the conversational partners of people of dementia that may compensate for the problems individuals with dementia encounter (Harré & van Langenhove, 1999).

The collaborative nature of communication implies that interlocutors may distribute interactional labour between them in interaction. From a dialogical perspective (Linell, 2009), where conversation is regarded as a collaborative project, conversations are seen as *joint activities*, implying that participants have some kind of shared goal, are committed to the activity, are mutually responsive to each other and also are mutually supportive (see also Tomasello, 2014). When people engage in a joint activity, each participant adds something new to the shared knowledge, the participants' common ground, and they shape the current state of their own activity (Clark, 1996, p. 58). Participants add something new through *contributions*, often in the form of spoken utterances, but sometimes also through gestures or an interactional package constituted by both verbal and nonverbal actions (see e.g. Goodwin, 2013). From an emergentist model of pragmatics (Perkins, 2007) and a dialogic perspective (Linell, 2009), interactants are responsive to each other, and through their own contributions they exhibit to each other how they understand one another and how they collaborate to divide interactional labour. The division of labour in interaction is assumed to be asymmetrical due to different knowledge, abilities and opportunities to participate in any communicative activity (Linell & Luckmann, 1991). Within this framework, pragmatic ability (which may be claimed to comprise collaboration in interaction) is composed of some basic principles that are used to motivate the model. First, pragmatics is claimed to involve a range of choices open to us in communication. Second, those choices can be made on different levels of processing and they may involve also the use of tools and artefacts as well as nonverbal resources in communication. The choices need to be motivated by the requirements of interpersonal communication and they may also be related to compensatory adaptations made by the participants in interaction, especially if one of the participants has communicative problems, such as in dementia (Perkins, 2007, pp. 51–52).

One way to compensate for communicative problems associated with dementia diseases is to change the division of contributions between the participants (see Hydén, 2014a, p. 117). By contributing more to the activity, being more responsible for the planning of the activity and engaging in repair work and helping to keep track of what has already been accomplished, communicative partners can engage in *scaffolding* of the person with dementia (ibid.; see also Hydén, 2011, 2014b; Müller & Mok, 2014). Through such scaffolding, the person with dementia is able to 'access those communicative and cognitive resources needed in order to continue participating in collaboration' (Hydén, 2014a, p. 117). The reorganization of communicative and cognitive resources as a strategy has been reported to be used also in relation to communication with people with other types of brain damage (e.g. Duff et al., 2012; Goodwin, 2003). This is in fact a compensatory strategy to solve communicative problems and may be equally adopted both by people with dementia and by their conversational partners. If, for example, the person with dementia has trouble remembering a name, he or she can either use an adaptive strategy himself or herself (e.g. a mnemonic technique) or be provided with the name by the interlocutor. In either way, the role of the conversational partner in providing support is crucial to the progression and the achievement of communicative activities.

In sum, interactionally oriented studies using a dialogical perspective on communication have shown us that collaboration is constituted by specific joint actions commonly observed in various types of activities. Collaboration is practiced through joint attention and negotiation of meaning (through verbal and nonverbal means) and providing scaffolding for people with dementia (see Hydén, 2014b) by the use of *feedback signals* (Hydén et al., 2013), attending to the repair initiations by people with dementia, using prompts, providing instructions and extra support in meaning-making practices and utilizing artefacts and tools in accomplishing activities (see Majlesi & Ekström, 2016, and Lindholm, 2013). In what follows, we will discuss some aspects of collaboration when encountering communicative problems in activities involving people with dementia in both institutional and everyday settings and how collaboration would help not only to solve the problems but also to keep people with dementia engaged in the current activity.

Collaboration in communication in daily activities

As discussed earlier, the ability to participate in any type of communicative activity may become limited for people with dementia when their cognitive and communicative abilities diminish. Depending on the stage of dementia, for a person with dementia to participate in everyday activities, it is often required that someone else both plan and monitor the activities (see e.g. Jansson et al., 2001). One of the main strategies used in collaboration with people with dementia is to provide support by engaging in talk and providing scaffolding (verbal and nonverbal resources) to accomplish the activity. Scaffolding may also involve assigning specific tasks formatted to fit a person's specific abilities, dividing a task into smaller and simpler subtasks and formulating and structuring tasks in correspondence to an individual's cognitive resources (cf. Vikström et al., 2008). In the following, we will discuss the details of such compensatory strategies and show the practical details of how collaborative communication with people with dementia may be organized and practised to the benefit of people with dementia as active participants in the activities in which they are involved.

Communication in care homes and day-care centres

Participating in interaction in institutional settings, like care homes and day-care centres, is challenging both for people with dementia and for their caregivers. The difficulties in communication are not only related to dementia but also to observable challenges in the context of communication. Some of these problems are caused by multiparty talk (more than two parties) where there is overlapping and parallel talk in interaction. Situations of overlapping talk easily create problems related to hearing and understanding (Drew, 1997), and parallel conversations can also be challenging to follow for people with dementia, who may have impaired skills in language production and comprehension, and in addition, hearing problems and attention deficits (Baddeley et al., 2001; Bayles & Tomoeda, 2007; Collette et al., 1999). This means that people with dementia recurrently encounter difficulties in group activities when caregivers speak to other participants without language and communication impairments (Lindholm, 2013). In addition, because of the diverse tasks of caregivers in institutional settings, they often need to perform other activities simultaneously while talking to the residents, and this easily results in hearing and comprehension problems (cf. Bayles & Tomoeda, 2007; Lindholm, 2013). Besides, institutional settings are often characterised by background noise and multiple concurrent stimuli, adding to the challenges experienced by people with dementia.

Residents in care homes and day-care centres usually have varying language and communication skills. This variation means that they differ in their abilities to participate in conversation. Caregivers may find it challenging when encouraging everyone to participate actively in group conversations and faced with situations in which some of the participants may withdraw from the interaction because of their communication difficulties. The differences in skills of the participants become evident in all kinds of conversations but are particularly prominent in certain activities, such as games (Lindholm, 2013). Providing an example from a game situation may illustrate how a caregiver at a day-care centre can compensate for the varying skills of the elderly persons as it actually happens when the conversation was recorded. In the example, Nurse Giselle is playing a type of bingo, using flowers instead of numbers, with three elderly participants: Anna, Olga and Ferdinand (all names are fictitious for ethical reasons). First, the nurse reads a description of a flower. Then the other participants try to guess the flower. Those who have the picture of the flower the nurse has described put a marker on their bingo cards. Anna has problems following the game and does not seem to be engaging. The nurse works actively to involve Anna in the game, through engaging her in conversation and thus compensating for Anna's difficulties.

Example 1: Aquavit.

```
01  Gis: what's [that
02  Ann:       [I was about to say aquavit ((to Olga))
03  Olg: that's aster th[en
04  Ann:              [but it does[n't fit in
05  Gis:                    [yes it's aster right ((to Olga))
06  Olg: yes
07  Gis: what were you going to say Anna (.hh) (0.2) aquavit?
08       (0.2)
09  Ann:  yes
10  Gis: [[heh heh[heh
11  Isa: [[heh heh[heh
12  Ann:         [*we're talking about* (0.2) *other things
                here*
```

In the example, the caregiver (Nurse Giselle) attends to a very farfetched playful guess that Anna makes (aquavit) and does not let her out of the game although her guess is not relevant to the game's domain. After she confirms Olga's guess about the flower, *aster*, in line 03, she engages in talk with Anna although Anna had not directly addressed Giselle when she made her guess (see line 02). Questioning someone's contribution in an activity is usually socially problematic as it may lead to social conflicts. Giselle's request for the repetition of Anna's response could thus be a potentially face-threatening act, because Anna's contribution to the ongoing activity may be seen as an exhibition of her inability to provide the searched-for response. However, it could also be regarded as a playful response. Anna's use of the past tense in line 02, *I **was** about to*, and her continuation in line 04, *but it doesn't fit in*, however, provide keys to interpreting that after all she had shown certain competence: she had considered giving the wrong answer, but she realized that it wouldn't fit in. Still, it remains a fact that Anna failed to provide the correct answer. However, Giselle provides an interactional space for Anna to put things right and she seems to be successful: the participants laugh together at Anna's suggestion, and Giselle manages to engage Anna in the activity.

Collaborating in communication and becoming a resource to help people with dementia may also be relevant to other participants with dementia, as they scaffold and help each other in group situations. In the following example, Ferdinand is telling about his experiences from World War II, explaining how the soldiers slept in tents. As a response to his telling, nurse Rebecka poses a question: *did you always have someone as a fire warden* (line 01). Rebecka's question causes Ferdinand problems, and David works actively with Rebecka to help Ferdinand grasp the message.

Example 2: Fire warden.

```
01  Reb: did you always have someone as a fire warden
02       (0.2)
03  Fer: what
04       (0.2)
05  Reb: did you always have someone who sat as a fire
         warden
06       (0.9)
07  Dav: <fire warden>
08       (1.6)
09  Reb: in [ta- in the tent
10  Dav:    [about that
11  Fer:       [I have a hearing problem
12  Dav: (about [that)
13  Reb:        [did someone always sit as a fire warden in
               the tent
14       (1.0)
15  Dav: did someone sit as a <fire warden>
16  Fer: yes yesyes yesyes (.h) *kipinäkalle*
17  Reb:  oh heh heh heh
```

As is obvious from the excerpt above, Ferdinand did not grasp what was asked by Rebecka (line 03) either because he did not understand Rebecka's question or, as he says (line 11), he has a hearing problem. When the repetition of the question does not help (line 05), David joins the conversation and concentrates on repeating the most important element of Rebecka's turn, *fire warden*, at a slower pace (line 07). When Ferdinand makes a second expression of his hearing problems (line 11), Rebecka repeats her previous question again (line 13). David, in his turn, assists Rebecka by reformulating her question (line 15), intensifying the articulation of *fire warden*, which is uttered slowly and with stress on the first syllable. In line 17, Ferdinand finally perceives what the others are talking about and responds by providing the Finnish element *kipinäkalle*, a playful expression for a fire warden, which may have been used by soldiers during World War II. It is impossible to say whether Ferdinand gains his new understanding as a result of only the previous repair turn or from the combined effect of several repair turns. However, Ferdinand is apparently helped by the combination of slower talk and repetitions of previous turns; the compensations provided by several co-participants, including a caregiver and another person with dementia, are successful.

As noted above, there are obvious difficulties related to interacting in institutional settings, caused by both the institutional environment and the impaired language and communication skills of the individuals. However, as the examples have shown, there are also opportunities to overcome these challenges. Group settings may provide opportunities for participants capable of collaborating and scaffolding each other and compensating for each other's shortcomings (Örulv, 2008; Lindholm, 2013). In line with the theory of emergent pragmatics, group conversations might thus function as a system where language and communication disorders 'become common property, rather than solely the problem of an individual' (Perkins, 2007, p. 67).

Communication in home environment: facilitating participation through instructions

Collaboration in any communicative activities is interactive by nature, and it might not be limited to providing verbal prompts but might also include helping a co-participant through instructed operations or tasks by, for example, providing embodied directives in hands-on activities (such as cooking, cleaning, etc.). Recently, it has been argued that providing *instructions* may be a way to collaborate and help people with dementia to participate in various everyday activities (Hydén, 2014a; Majlesi & Ekström, 2016; Ekström & Majlesi, forthcoming). Providing instructions in face-to-face ordinary interaction is usually concomitant with a constant supply of directives and requests (see e.g. Goodwin & Cekaite, 2013). Telling someone else what to do can be done in a number of different ways, including orders, commands, assignments, requests, suggestions, proposals and hints (e.g. Ervin-Trapp, 1976; Searle, 1979; Stevanovic & Svennevig, 2015). The kind of directive used in a certain situation displays to what degree the speaker 'assumes control over the recipient's actions', and 'the very fact that so many different ways of "getting someone to do something" exist, highlights the careful negotiation that can be required when initiating an action that impinges on another person's freedom of action' (Kent, 2012, p. 712). While directives have been foregrounded as key to both controlling and eliciting actions of another party (Ervin-Trapp, 1976), it can also be a resource to facilitate a person with dementia participating in ongoing activities (Hydén,

2014a; Jansson et al., 2001; Majlesi & Ekström, 2016; Vikström et al., 2005, 2008). Giving directives can be initiated by the co-interactants of a person with dementia or in the response to the request by the person with dementia. In a recent study, it has been argued that directives 'provide an interactional environment wherein the person with dementia can make contributions to the joint activity in an efficient way' (Majlesi & Ekström, 2016, p. 44). Activities organised around directive sequences are described as 'interactional environments where the person with dementia may be given opportunities to actively exhibit his/her abilities and knowledge in accomplishing the given tasks and participate in everyday activities' (ibid. 45).

Several studies have shown that the ways directives are designed are contingent on to whom the request is being made and in what context (e.g. Antaki & Kent, 2012; Goodwin & Cekaite, 2013; Craven & Potter, 2010; Curl & Drew, 2008; Heinemann, 2006; Lindström, 2007; Mondada, 2014). Generally, in ordinary, adult-adult interaction, entitled directives are considered to be an invasive, and sometimes even offensive, action (Brown & Levinson, 1987). While directives among (adult) friends are often both mitigated and delayed (as in the form of requests), in task-oriented activities as well as in parent-child interaction, directives are neither delayed nor oriented towards as troublesome but rather are a basic resource through which the activities are accomplished (Goodwin & Cekaite, 2013). This seems also to be the case in interaction involving people with dementia. For example, in interaction between people with dementia and their family caregivers at home environments, directives have been shown to be produced without hesitation or other mitigating actions (Ekström & Majlesi, forthcoming). In their study of a couple living with dementia, Ekström and Majlesi (forthcoming) show that directives seem to be recurrently formulated as telling the person with dementia what to do, as opposed to, for example, asking or suggesting an action for the person with dementia (cf. various forms of directive in Ervin-Trapp, 1976). As shown in their study, neither the caregiver nor the person with dementia orients towards giving directives as interactionally problematic but rather as an expected routine action in the activities.

The examples below show parts of the collaboration between a couple, Ellen and her husband, Tom, who is diagnosed with middle-stage Alzheimer's disease, when they are doing various kitchen chores. The directives are either initiated by Ellen or emerge in response to Tom's inquiries.

Example 3: Unplugging.

```
01   Tom: ((turns off the water))
02   (7.7)((puts the pot on the countertop and takes out
     a dishtowel))
03   Ell: can you unplugg that one there, then,
04        (0.6)
```

```
05  Tom: is this a dish towel? this one or is it ((holds
         a dish towel))
06  Ell: yeah that's a dish towel
07  (1.3)
08  Ell: °(m)° (0.2) you can unplugg that one there,
09  (1.1) ((Tom puts down a bowl and leans toward the cord))
10  Ell: when you have it (.) taken away=
11  Tom: =that?
12  Ell: yeah
13  (1.0) ((Tom unpluggs the dough maker))
14  Ell: that one should (0.2) should be put away
15       ((Tom does what was asked him to do))
```

In collaborative activities involving people with dementia, as the example above shows, instructions are usually set out by the caregiver through a series of directives. Ellen monitors how Tom accomplishes the tasks and if necessary, comes in with extra guidance to help Tom with further instructions. She is also aware of providing the next task only when the previous one is fulfilled. In this way, she manages to keep Tom participating in what is constructed as a joint activity in the kitchen, and she also controls the flow of the tasks in the kitchen. The example is evidence that collaboration does not mean that mutuality and commonality as the indispensible feature of communication may necessarily entail equal roles, knowledge and opportunities of participants in a communicative activity (Linell & Luckmann, 1991). Sometimes mutuality and reciprocities are mirrored in the social actions (such as greeting) and sometimes they vary and in fact become 'complementary' in social relations (ibid, p. 3; e.g. giving instructions and following them). Thus, collaboration may entail asymmetrical division of labour both in terms of being responsible for activities with various difficulties and in terms of providing directives and assuming rights and entitlements to instruct.

Scaffolding in joint activities with people with dementia: elaborating on some compensatory strategies

So far, we have discussed a dialogical approach (Linell, 2009) together with an emergent pragmatic perspective (Perkins, 2007) to communicative activities involving people with dementia, where we also demonstrated through examples how such activities require certain collaborative actions by both parties in terms of compensatory strategies. In what follows, we will attend to some aspects of such collaboration, and particularly the strategy of task division to facilitate the participation of people with dementia in social activities, especially multitask everyday activities. We will emphasise the significance of embodiment in interaction with people with dementia and will also show the mutuality in collaboration by attending to the specific compensatory strategy used by people with dementia in exploiting their communicative partner as a resource in interaction.

Sequencing and the use of subtasks

In collaborative activities involving people with dementia, scaffolding in the form of the guiding actions of the co-participants are largely oriented towards what might be called structuring work. Instructions and other guiding actions are mainly directed towards providing information about what task should be performed next (Hydén, 2014a; Majlesi & Ekström, 2016). This generally divides the activity in subtasks and sequences these subtasks in a particular order. Focusing on smaller subtasks and performing one task at a time facilitates the participation of people with dementia in the activity (see Hydén, 2014a).

In the following example, the same couple as in Example 3 are baking cinnamon buns. It is time to coat buns with egg and sugar, and Ellen assigns this task to her husband, Tom, diagnosed with dementia. Ellen is not only dividing the main activity (coating the buns) into smaller subtasks, but she is also separating these subtasks into smaller and more manageable units.

Example 4: Preparing eggs.

```
01   Ell: (we)'re going to prepare the egg so (then) you
          can bring those
02        things
03        (1.3)
04   Tom: are we going to use this? ((holds a plastic can
          in front of Ellen))
05        (0.2)
06   Ell: yeah
07        (1.6)
08   Ell: (you prepare) (.) you can prepare two eggs at once
```

Having introduced the first sub-activity (preparing the eggs), Ellen directs Tom to 'get those things' (line 01). Tom is already standing next to the cupboard where the things needed to prepare the eggs are stored, something that might help him grasp which things Ellen is referring to and where to find them. When Tom has found the right items and Ellen has confirmed that they are, indeed, the things she was asking for, Ellen continues by telling Tom to prepare two eggs at once (line 08). While this statement is not designed as a reminder of what the main task is, but merely as an additional instruction on the number of eggs to prepare, the instruction nevertheless functions as a prompt for Tom to continue with the activity and a cue for what to do next (fetch the eggs). Tom walks to the fridge and after some discussion with Ellen on the size of the eggs, he fetches two eggs and both cracks and shakes them without Ellen telling him to do so. While instructions are both important and sometimes necessary to facilitate the actions for a person with dementia, it can be equally important to withhold instructions when they are not required. Performing small tasks independently and without a preceding directive from a caregiver could be beneficial for a person's self-esteem and selfhood.

As previously argued by Hydén (2014a), dividing a task into smaller subtasks and providing a structure that sequences these subtasks seems to be a fruitful way to organize an activity where a person with dementia can not only participate but also make important contributions to the overall activity. The caregiver in the example above guides and supports the person with dementia, but, at the same time, she leaves room for him to initiate actions and to perform parts of the tasks independently when suitable.

Embodied guidance and nonverbal communication

Collaboration and compensatory strategies through guiding and instructing people with dementia may involve not only verbal directives but can also be constituted by nonverbal actions. In relation to people with dementia, this could be especially fruitful as nonverbal instructions – such as demonstrations (Lindwall & Ekström, 2012), showing where things are by pointing (Mondad, 2014), or even using shepherding action (Cekaite, 2010) – can effectively guide the person with dementia's focus, perception and orientations in the activity. While touch is recurrently used between couples living with dementia as in the following case, it goes without saying that it should be used with care and consideration of respecting one's personal space.

Following the same couple in the example below, we present a sequence of events during which Ellen suggests that it is coffee time (line 01), and instructs Tom with a directive to sit down first by pointing to a place 'here' (line 03) and then by actually guiding him bodily towards a chair (line 04). Tom complies with the request both verbally and with the actual performance of the instruction (line 05).

Example 5: Coffee time.

```
01  Ell: we could need some (.) coffee
02       (5)
03  Tom: a:
```

```
04   Ell: you can sit down here then Tom ((pointing toward
          a chair and
05        touching Tom on the arm in a guiding action
          toward the chair))
06   Tom: yes then I do that ((Tom walks toward the
          appointed chair))
07   Ell: this one (.) I've been meaning to ask you if
          you've seen this (1)
08        this have you seen this one ((fetches a maga-
          zine and shows to Tom,
09        who is now standing beside the kitchen table))
10        (1)
10   Ell: sit down and have a [look ((hands over the
          magazine to Tom))
11   Tom:               [yeah::
```

This example shows that collaboration may require embodied engagement in the activity and helping people with dementia using hands-on practices. Providing directives as a strategy to get a person to do something may also involve *embodied directives*, that is, instructional directives that are constituted both by talk and by visible display of embodied ways of performing the tasks (e.g. pointing and touching). Although Ellen's monitoring and instructing through embodied directives may be inferred as exerting social control over the activity of the person with dementia, Ellen's actions could also be considered as scaffolding resources. Through her doings, Ellen provides opportunities for Tom to be engaged in the activity, and to do so in an efficient way. Participating even in a seemingly simple practice of having coffee, considering the condition of the person with dementia, requires certain skills and competencies, and through her instructional actions, Ellen provides Tom with the sufficient support to be able to participate in this activity.

People with dementia as competent collaborative partners

Several studies (Hydén, 2014a; Hydén et al., forthcoming; Majlesi & Ekström, 2016) show that people with dementia not only are able to participate in – and contribute to – collaborative activities, they even participate in skilful, independent ways when they are provided with a sequential structure that temporally links the various subtasks into an overall activity. Dementia seems to mainly affect overall organisational skills and not to the same extent the abilities to perform practical, everyday tasks (naturally depending on the severity of the condition). This is, for instance, indicated by the kind of instructions given to people with dementia in collaborative joint activities. In collaborative joint activities, instructions usually do not include the reason for doing a specific task, and the specific procedures involved in performing a task are also often treated as already known. This may indicate that the practices and procedures involved in carrying out various everyday tasks and activities are not expected to be affected by a dementia disease.

While the work caregivers and relatives do is essential to facilitate the participation of people with dementia, it is important not to overlook the compensatory strategies used by people with dementia themselves to manage difficulties and problems in communication. Several studies have demonstrated how people with dementia can actively use the material environment – including collaborating partners – to compensate for challenges they encounter (e.g. Hydén, 2014a; Majlesi & Ekström, 2016). Collaborators definitely play an important role for people with dementia to be able to participate in everyday activities, but recent studies indicate that people with dementia are much more active in the accomplishment of collaborative activities than has previously been described (ibid). While collaborating partners usually need to take on responsibilities for initiating activities and guiding people with dementia, people with dementia are also actively seeking the guidance and support they need to be able to accomplish the task at hand. People with dementia may use various methods when faced with difficulties in interaction. In what follows, we will brief out some of the problems and corresponding solutions used in interaction to overcome various difficulties.

Soliciting help and initiating repair

As shown in the examples above, people with dementia recurrently, like any other communicative partners, ask their collaborator questions as a way to obtain information. This could, for example, be a repair initiation to understand the request (Example 6, line 03) or a solicitation for help in doing or finding something (Example 7, line 08).

Example 6.

```
01  Ell:  (then) you fetch the pearl sugar then
02           (0.4)
03  Tom:  >what?<
```

Example 7.

```
08  Tom:  °where did I put it now°=
09  Ell:  =no you haven't got that °yet°
```

While repeatedly asking a partner for information might be seen as an indication of *inability*, a more fruitful way to understand the asking of questions might be to see this as a strategy to compensate for (perceived) inabilities and thereby show *competence* in solving the emerging problems in interaction (seeing it dialogically, Linell, 2009). By asking questions, people with dementia not only show that they are aware of what they need to know in order to continue the activity at hand and that they recognise how to get this information (Lindholm, 2014); they also competently avoid doing things that might generate mistakes by asking for further instructions when the instructions given are not adequate to act on.

Seeking confirmation and validation

As mentioned above, seeking confirmation could be a practice for people with dementia to also receive validation from their collaborating partners when making contributions to the joint activities (e.g. following the instructions). In collaborative activities, people with dementia have been seen to frequently ask their collaborating partner to confirm and validate their actions and choices and to help decide when a subtask is properly and adequately performed (Majlesi & Ekström, 2016). This kind of confirmation seeking is done both orally, by asking the partner, and by showing the results of choices and actions to the partner. Similar to the practice of asking questions, recurrent confirmation seeking is used as a compensatory strategy by people with dementia. Although it could also be viewed as a sign of incompetence and inability in relation to the current activity, this kind of behaviour can also signal a skilled strategy to avoid making mistakes. In this sense, the person with dementia can be seen to actively use his or partner as a compensatory resource in the accomplishment of the task.

The following example demonstrates such a practice. When preparing eggs for baking cinnamon buns (Examples 8 and 9), Ellen introduces the task of preparing eggs and suggests that they are going to brush the eggs over the buns. Then she provides a directive to Tom to fetch a can to use for mixing the eggs:

Example 8: Preparing eggs.

```
01  Ell: (we)'re going to prepare the egg so (then) you
         can bring those
02       things
03       (1.3)
04  Tom: are we going to use this? ((holds a plastic can
         in front of Ellen))
05               (0.2)
06  Ell: yeah
```

In the unfolding interaction, Tom demonstrates his competence in understanding what Ellen means by the word 'stuff' (line 01) in the first place. However, Tom seeks confirmation to match the indexical expression with what he took out of the cupboard. He holds a plastic can in front of Ellen and asks *'are we going to use this?'* (line 04). In this way, he categorically knows he was in the right and Ellen confirms it in her response (line 06).

Verbalizing and commenting on an ongoing action

Another, more subtle, practice used by people with dementia, which also functions as a strategy to avoid making mistakes, is *online commentaries* accompanying their own actions (Majlesi & Ekström, 2016). When participating in collaborative activities, people with dementia sometimes describe their own actions aloud but without specifically addressing their collaborators (Lindholm, 2016). While the motive behind this kind of behaviour is not possible to discern without speculations, one function it plays in collaborative activities is to make it possible for collaborating partners to follow and monitor – and thereby if necessary also correct – the actions of the person with dementia. The following example shows a sample of such online commentaries and how Ellen, the family caregiver of Tom, responds to those comments by giving reassurance as to the correctness of his actions. It is an excerpt of an activity in which Tom is putting the electric mixer away, and he has to rearrange things in the cupboard to make a place for the mixer.

Example 9.

```
01   Ell: and then you put (.) can't have that one in
          there no put [it away
02        down there
03   Tom:                              [those]
04        I put in there
05   Ell: yeah that's right
06        (1.0)
07   Tom: [(like that)]
08   Ell: [and] then [(you have to)-]
09   Tom: °(that one goes)° (0.3) °(here)°
10        (2.6) ((Tom puts away the dough maker in the
          cupboard))
11   Ell: there you go (.) perfect
```

As the example shows, when Tom receives the directives as to how to rearrange things in the cupboard (line 01), he verbalizes what he does in his response (lines 02 and 03). He does it without looking at Ellen. Tom's action, however, is positively and affirmatively responded to by Ellen (line 04). When Tom continues to comment further on his own action (line 08), again Ellen provides feedback on his comment and confirms his action (line 10).

In the example, Tom makes available his own actions to his collaborating partner through verbal formulations of his doing. In this way, he provides his partner with the opportunity to follow, adjust and correct his performance in the current task. Careful observations of communication with people with dementia would reveal strategies that can be used to benefit people with dementia by helping them successfully participate in interaction and accomplish the task or the activity in which they are engaged.

Conclusion

In this chapter, we have introduced two closely related perspectives on communication (Linell, 1998; Perkins, 1997) and discussed how these perspectives can be used to adjust understandings of dementia and communication in a way that emphasises communicative abilities of people rather than communicative problems. In the chapter, we have argued for the importance of viewing communication as a collaborative activity, in which participants are mutually and cooperatively responsible for meaning making and understanding. Using examples from various contexts, we have demonstrated the significance of using an integrated approach in which verbal and nonverbal communicative resources are understood as mutually supporting and co-dependent systems working together when conveying meaning (Goodwin, 2007; Heath & Hindmarsh, 2002; Streeck et al., 2011). In the chapter, we have put forward *collaboration* as a way to increase the engagement of people with dementia and examined how communicative activities can be organised to facilitate people with dementia participating in and contributing to various communicative activities. We have also introduced the concept of *scaffolding* (Hydén, 2014a; see also Hydén, 2011, 2014b; Müller & Mok, 2014) as a way to compensate for communicative problems associated with dementia diseases. By changing the division of contributions between the participants towards an increased responsibility for communicative partners, people with dementia can gain access to information and resources that are no longer readily available to them.

While caregivers – both formal and informal – constitute invaluable support to guarantee that people with dementia continue to participate in communicative activities, we have also underlined the importance of not portraying people with dementia as passive receivers of guidance and support. Through our examples, we have demonstrated a number of compensatory strategies used by people with dementia themselves (Hydén, 2014a; Lindholm, 2013, 2014; Majlesi & Ekström, 2016; Örulv, 2008). People with dementia have been shown to scaffold each other and share the responsibilities for problems that occur (Lindholm,

2013; Örulv, 2008; cf. Perkins, 2007), and they are also actively pursuing the support they need to be able to accomplish a current activity. In the chapter, we have shown examples in which people with dementia are not only aware of what kind of information they need and how to get this information – they also competently use strategies to avoid doing things that might generate mistakes. The described collection of compensatory strategies, along with the dialogical and emergentist theoretical views (Linell, 1998; Perkins, 1997), are of great clinical relevance. Enhancing the active participation of people with dementia, and viewing their actions from a dialogical perspective, will have an impact on their possibilities of maintaining their identity as competent and active participants in the society.

References

Alm, N., Astell, A., Ellis, M., Dye, R., Gowans, G. & Campbell, J. (2004). A cognitive prosthesis and communication support for people with dementia. *Neuropsychological Rehabilitation, 14*, 117–134.

Almor, A., Kempler, D., MacDonald, M., Andersen, E. & Tyler, L. (1999). Why do Alzheimer patients have difficulty with pronouns? Working memory, semantics, and reference in comprehension and production in Alzheimer's disease. *Brain and Language, 67*, 202–227.

Antaki, C. & Kent, A. (2012). Telling people what to do (and, sometimes, why): Contingency, entitlement and explanation in staff requests to adults with intellectual impairments. *Journal of Pragmatics, 44*, 876–889.

Azuma, T. & Bayles, K. A. (1997). Memory impairments underlying language difficulties in dementia. *Topics in Language Disorders, 18*, 58–71.

Baddeley, A. D., Baddeley, H. A., Bucks, R. S. & Wilcock, G. K. (2001). Attentional control in Alzheimer's disease. *Brain, 124*, 1492–1508.

Bayles, K. A. & Tomoeda, C. K. (2007). *Cognitive-Communication Disorders of Dementia.* San Diego, CA: Plural Publishing.

Bayles, K. A., Tomoeda, C. K., Kaszniak, A. W., Stern, L. Z. & Eagans, K. K. (1985). Verbal perseveration of dementia patients. *Brain and Language, 25*, 102–116.

Brown, P. & Levinson, S. (1987). *Politeness: Some Universals in Language Usage.* Cambridge: Cambridge University Press.

Causino Lamar, M. A., Obler, L. K., Knoefel, J. E. & Albert, M. L. (1995). Communication patterns in end-stage Alzheimer's disease: Pragmatic analysis. In R. L. Bloom, L. K. Obler, S. de Santi & J. S. Ehrlich (Eds.), *Discourse Analysis and Applications: Studies in Adult Clinical Populations* (pp. 217–235). Hillsdale, NJ: Lawrence Erlbaum Associates.

Cekaite, A. (2010). Shepherding the child: Embodied directive sequences in parent-child interactions. *Text & Talk-An Interdisciplinary Journal of Language, Discourse & Communication Studies, 30*(1), 1.

Clare, L. (2008). *Neuropsychological Rehabilitation and People with Dementia.* New York: Psychology Press.

Craven, A. & Potter, J. (2010). Directives: Entitlement and contingency in action. *Discourse Studies, 12*, 419–442.

Clark, H. H. (1996). *Using Language.* New York: Cambridge University Press.

Collette, F., van der Linden, M., Salmon, E. & Bechet, S. (1999). Phonological loop and central executive functioning in Alzheimer's disease. *Neuropsychologia, 37*, 905–918.

Curl, T. S. & Drew, P. (2008). Contingency and action: A comparison of two forms of requesting. *Research on Language and Social Interaction, 41*, 129–153.

Drew, P. (1997). 'Open'class repair initiators in response to sequential sources of troubles in conversation. *Journal of Pragmatics, 28*(1), 69–101.

Duff, M. C., Mutlu, B., Byom, L. & Turkstra, L. S. (2012). Beyond utterances: Distributed cognition as a framework for studying discourse in adults with acquired brain injury. *Seminars in Speech and Language, 33*, 44–54.

Dunn, L. A., Rout, U., Carson, J. & Ritter, S. A. (1994). Occupational stress amongst care staff working in nursing homes: An empirical investigation. *Journal of Clinical Nursing, 3*, 177–183.

Ericsson, I., Hellstrom, I. & Kjellström, S. (2011). Sliding interactions: An ethnography about how persons with dementia interact in housing with care for the elderly. *Dementia, 10*, 523–538.

Ervin-Trapp, S. (1976). Is Sybil there? The structure of some American English directives. *Language in Society, 5*, 25–66.

Evans, S., Fear, T., Means, R. & Vallelly, S. (2007). Supporting independence for people with dementia in extra care housing. *Dementia, 6*, 144–150.

Goodwin, C. (2003). *Conversation and Brain Damage.* Oxford: Oxford University Press.

Goodwin, C. (2007). Environmentally coupled gestures. In S. D. Duncan, J. Cassell & E. T. Levy (Eds.), *Gesture and the Dynamic Dimension of Language* (pp. 195–212). Amsterdam & Philadelphia: John Benjamins Publishing Company.

Goodwin, C. (2013). The co-operative, transformative organization of human action and knowledge. *Journal of Pragmatics, 46*(1), 8–23.

Goodwin, M. H. & Cekaite, A. (2013). Calibration in directive-response trajectories in family interactions. *Journal of Pragmatics, 46*, 122–138.

Guendouzi, J. A. & Müller, N. (2006). *Approaches to Discourse in Dementia.* Mahwah, NJ : Lawrence Erlbaum Associates.

Hamilton, H. E. (1994). *Conversations with an Alzheimer's Patient. An Interactional Sociolinguistic Study.* Cambridge: Cambridge University Press.

Harré, R. & Van Langenhove, L. (1999). The dynamics of social episodes. In R. Harré & L. van Langenhove (Eds.), *Positioning Theory* (pp. 1–13). Oxford: Blackwell Publisher Ltd.

Heath, C. & Hindmarsh, J. (2002). Analysing interaction: Video, ethnography and situated conduct. In T. May (Ed.), *Qualitative Rresearch in Practice* (pp. 99–121). London: Sage.

Heinemann, T. (2006). 'Will you or can't you?': Displaying entitlement in interrogative requests, *Journal of Pragmatics, 38*, 1081–1104.

Hydén, L.-C. (2011). Narrative collaboration and scaffolding in dementia. *Journal of Aging Studies, 25*, 339–347.

Hydén, L. C. (2014a). Cutting Brussels sprouts: Collaboration involving persons with dementia. *Journal of Aging Studies, 29*, 115–123.

Hydén, L. C. (2014b). How to do things with others: Joint activities involving persons with Alzheimer's disease. In L. C. Hydén, H. Lindemann & J. Brockmeier (Eds.), *Beyond Loss: Dementia, Identity, and Personhood* (pp. 137–154). New York: Oxford University Press.

Hydén, L. C. (in press). *Entangled Narratives:Collaborative Storytelling and the Re-Imagining of Dementia.* New York: Oxford University Press.

Hydén, L. C., Plejert, C. Samuelsson, C. & Örulv, L. (2013). Feedback and common ground in conversational storytelling involving people with Alzheimer's disease. *Journal of Interactional Research in Communication Disorders, 4*, 211–247.

Jansson, W., Nordberg, G. & Grafström, M. (2001). Patterns of elderly spousal caregiving in dementia care: An observational study. *Journal of Advanced Nursing, 34*, 804–812.

Kent, A. (2012). Compliance, resistance and incipient compliance when responding to directives. *Discourse Studies, 14*(6), 711–730.

Kitwood, T. (1997). *Dementia Reconsidered: The Person Comes First.* Buckingham: Open University Press.

Lindholm, C. (2013). Challenges and opportunities of group conversations: The day care center as a communication milieu. In B. H. Davis & J. Guendouzi (Eds.), *Pragmatics in Dementia Discourse* (pp. 205–238). Cambridge: Cambridge Scholars Publishing.

Lindholm, C. (2014). Comprehension in interaction: Communication at a day care center. In L.C. Hydén, J. Brockmeier & H. Lindemann (Eds.), *Beyond Loss: Dementia, Identity, Personhood* (pp. 155–172). Oxford: Oxford University Press.

Lindholm, C. (2016). Boundaries of participation in care home settings: The use of the Swedish token jaså by a person with dementia. *Clinical Linguistics and Phonetics,* 832–848. doi:10.1080/02699206.2016.1208275

Lindström, A. (2007). Language as social action: A study of how senior citizens request assistance with practical tasks in the Swedish home help service. In A. Hakulinen & M. Selting (Eds.), *Syntax and Lexis in Conversation: Studies on the Use of Linguistic Resources in Talk-in-Interaction* (pp. 209–230). Amsterdam & Philadelphia: John Benjamins Publishing Company.

Lindwall, O. & Ekström, A. (2012). Instruction-in-interaction: The teaching and learning of a manual skill. *Human Studies, 35*, 27–49.

Linell, P. (1998). *Approaching Dialogue: Talk, Interaction and Contexts in Dialogical Perspectives* (Vol. 3). Amsterdam: John Benjamins Publishing.

Linell, P. (2009). *Rethinking Language, Mind, and World Dialogically: Interactional and Contextual Theories of Human Sense-making.* Charlotte, NC.: Information Age Publishing.

Linell, P., & Luckmann, T. (1991). Asymmetries in dialogue: some conceptual preliminaries. *Asymmetries in Dialogue,* 1–20.

Majlesi, A. R. & Ekström, A. (2016). Baking together – the coordination of actions in activities involving people with dementia. *Journal of Aging Studies, 38*, 37–46.

Maxim, J. & Bryan, K. (2006). Language, communication and cognition in the dementias. In K. Bryan & J. Maxim (Eds.), *Communication Disability in the Dementias* (pp. 73–124). London: Whurr Publishers.

Mondada, L. (2014). Instructions in the operating room: How the surgeon directs their assistant's hands. *Discourse Studies, 16*, 131–161.

Murphy, J., Oliver, T. M. & Cox, S. (2010). *Talking Mats and Involvement in Decision Making for People with Dementia and Family Carers.* Joseph Rowntree Foundation.

Müller, N. & Mok, Z. (2014). 'Getting to know you': Situated and distributed cognition in conversation with dementia. In R. W. Schrauf & N. Müller (Eds.), *Dialogue and Dementia: Cognitive and Communicative Resources for Engagement* (pp. 61–86). New York: Psychology Press.

Örulv, L. (2008). *Fragile identities, patched-up worlds: Dementia and meaning-making in social interaction.* PhD dissertation, Linköping University Electronic Press.

Örulv, L. & Hydén, L. C. (2006). Confabulation: Sense-making, self-making and world-making in dementia. *Discourse Studies, 8*, 647–673.

Örulv, L. & Nikku, N. (2007). Dignity work in dementia care: Sketching a microethical analysis. *Dementia, 6*, 507–525.

Perkins, M. (2007). *Pragmatic Impairment*. Cambridge: Cambridge University Press.

Perkins, L., Whitworth, A. & Lesser, R. (1998). Conversing in dementia: A conversation analytic approach. *Journal of Neurolinguistics, 11*, 33–53.

Ramanathan, V. (1997). *Alzheimer Discourse. Some Sociolinguistic Dimensions*. Mahwah, NJ: Lawrence Erlbaum Associates.

Ramanathan-Abbott, V. (1994). Interactional differences in Alzheimer's discourse: An examination of AD speech across two audiences. *Language in Society, 23*, 31–58.

Ripich, D. N. & Terrell, B. Y. (1988). Patterns of discourse cohesion and coherence in Alzheimer's disease. *Journal of Speech and Hearing Disorders, 53*, 8–19.

Sabat, S. (1991). Turn-taking, turn-giving and Alzheimer's disease: A case study in conversation. *Georgetown Journal of Language and Linguistics, 2*, 161–175.

Sabat, S. R. (1994). Recognizing and working with remaining abilities: Toward improving the care of Alzheimer's disease suffers. *The American Journal of Alzheimer's Care and Related Disorders & Research, 9*, 8–16.

Sabat, S. R. (2002). Surviving manifestations of selfhood in Alzheimer's disease: A case study. *Dementia, 1*, 25–36.

Sacks, H., Schegloff, E. A. & Jefferson, G. (1974). A simplest systematics for the organization of turn-taking for conversation. *Language, 50*, 696–735.

Saunders, P. A., de Medeiros, K., Doyle, P. & Mosby, A. (2012). The discourse of friendship: Mediators of communication among dementia residents in long-term care. *Dementia, 12*, 347–361.

Schegloff, E. A. (1987). Analyzing single episodes of interaction: An exercise in conversation analysis. *Social Psychology Quarterly*, 101–114.

Schulz, R. & O'Brien, A. T. (1994). Alzheimer's disease caregiving: An overview. *Seminars in Speech and Language, 15*, 185–194.

Searle, J. R. (1979). *Expression and Meaning: Studies in the Theory of Speech Acts*. Cambridge: Cambridge University Press.

Stevanovic, M. & Svennevig, J. (2015). Introduction: Epistemics and deontics in conversational directives. *Journal of Pragmatics, 78*, 1–6.

Streeck, J., Goodwin, C. & LeBaron, C. (2011). *Embodied Interaction: Language and Body in the Material World*. New York: Cambridge University Press.

Tomasello, M. (2014). *A Natural History of Human Thinking*. Cambridge: Harvard University Press.

Vikström, S., Borell, L., Stigsdotter-Neely, A. & Josephsson, S. (2005). Caregivers' self-initiated support towards their spouses with dementia when performing an everyday occupation together at home. *OTJR: Occupation, Participation and Health, 25*, 149–159.

Vikström, S., Josephsson, S., Stigsdotter-Neely, A. & Nygard, L. (2008). Engagement in activities: Experiences of persons with dementia and their caregiving spouses. *Dementia, 7*, 251–270.

Williamson, G. M. & Schulz, R. (1993). Coping with specific stressors in Alzheimer's disease caregiving. *The Gerontologist, 33*, 747–755.

Wright, L. W. (1993). *Alzheimer's Disease and Marriage*. Newbury Park, CA: Sage Publications.

7

STORYTELLING IN DEMENTIA: COLLABORATION AND COMMON GROUND

Lars-Christer Hydén

Stories are told everywhere by everyone. Everyday talk as well as talk at work is full of small conversational stories detailing events and experiences, as well as longer stories told to friends, family and colleagues. One reason stories are ubiquitous in everyday life is that they have important social functions. Telling stories is a way to share experiences and various perspectives on events and thus to create increased social coherence in relations (Mandelbaum, 1987). Stories also have a central role for people to present and negotiate their identities, both individual and collective ones (Kellas, 2005). It is thus reasonable to argue that the ability to take active part in storytelling activities is fundamental to most people. This implies that losing this ability can be problematic, even challenging the social and psychological status of the person and relations with other people.

Dementia is often a long process spread out over many years, and the person with dementia changes profoundly in the process: from being a person who experiences just minor functional changes in cognitive and linguistic resources, to a person at the late stages of dementia with very few resources available. The argument in this chapter is that storytelling is still a relevant activity for the person with dementia throughout all these different stages for the simple reason that both the person with dementia and other family members have much of their identity invested in everyday stories, and they all continue to tell stories even when the person with dementia has severe problems with animating the stories. As the dementia progresses, there are changes in patterns of engagement of the person with dementia in the storytelling activity. What is typical for storytelling involving persons with dementia is the fact that the storyteller is affected by the disease. Some persons with dementia can tell autobiographical stories on their own, while others can do it with support, especially from their spouses. Some persons with dementia tell autobiographical stories that leave the listener with a sense of confusion as their stories are often fragmented and repetitive; others repeat the same story over and over again or never find the words and abandon the story; sometimes gestures become more prominent than words.

Dementia affects the common ground between people, that is, what a person can take for granted that the other knows. Some of the common ground between people consists of their shared experiences and memories. As dementia affects memory, this common ground will be challenged. As a result, telling stories and presenting identities will become much more complicated and lead to a change in the relations between the person with dementia and significant others. For the person with dementia, as well as for the significant others, there is a need to deal with this changing common ground because otherwise joint storytelling will become impossible.

A central question in this chapter is whether it is possible to identify ways for persons with dementia to sustain participation in storytelling and hence to keep identity and social status. This chapter is an attempt not only to point to a number of strategies but also to introduce a theoretical framework that will allow an understanding of storytelling in dementia.

There are four important caveats. First, the focus of this chapter is on persons with dementia telling stories – not others telling stories about persons with dementia or others constructing life stories about persons with dementia. Thus there is no discussion about life-story work or other similar techniques used in care work with persons with dementia (for a review, see McKeown et al., 2006).

Second, this chapter is about good examples and the working ways people living with dementia have found and use. It is not about failures and lost opportunities.

Third, it is not about the stories told by persons with dementia – but about *the storytelling activity*. The reason is that although dementia might involve illness stories about dementia, the impact of dementia primarily has to do with the changes of the storyteller as a storytelling subject. As a consequence of this, the focus is on the activity of telling stories and about how dementia affects participation in this activity and how these changes affect the person and relations to others. A central idea in this chapter is that the storytelling activity is part of a wider social psychological web of relations between persons: their relations as well as not only their individual identities but also their shared identities. So looking at stories and storytelling is looking at how relations between persons are affected by dementia.

Fourth, for reasons of simplicity, this chapter mainly finds its examples among spouses living together telling stories about their shared lives. It is hoped that the introduced model of collaborative storytelling involving persons with dementia can be used also in other types of constellations of storytelling. Of special interest, of course, are care situations involving care professionals who work with the same person with dementia over many years. Together they will hopefully develop a relation that can be similar to spouses living together in at least one respect: they share a growing common ground. This common ground is different from the spouses' in that it is at least partially asymmetric: the person with dementia will know less about the professional nurse than the nurse will know about the person with dementia. Although this difference is important, many of the challenges that nurses and persons with dementia face in care settings are not that different from the challenges spouses will encounter in the context of their home.

In this chapter, a model of storytelling involving persons with dementia is introduced, consisting of four elements (for a more comprehensive discussion of storytelling and dementia, see Hydén, 2017):

- The first element is that all storytelling is *collaborative*, that is, all participants in this joint activity – whether they are listeners or tellers – must collaborate in order to engage with the same story.

- The second element is the concept of *common ground*. Part of telling a story is the use and creation of common ground, that is, knowledge pertinent to the story that all participants can assume and expect the others to have.

- The third element is the notion of the *fragmentation* and *redefinition of the common ground*. As a consequence of Alzheimer's disease in particular, the person will be challenged in using the common ground, and thus storytelling about shared events will become increasingly problematic.

- The fourth element has to do with the *compensatory strategies* that the participants in storytelling events can use in order for the person with dementia to continue as a participant. Of particular interest is what is called *collaborative compensatory adaptions*, for instance *scaffolding* strategies.

Storytelling as collaboration

Much research on dementia and storytelling has focused on the individual and his or her abilities to tell a 'coherent' and 'true' autobiographical story. Against this, it could be argued that storytelling is typically a joint activity engaging at least two persons who collaborate. This indicates a need for a theoretical framework for describing and understanding joint activities and collaboration involving persons with dementia. Steps in this theoretical direction have already been taken by a number of researchers on dementia, from Gubrium's early work (1986) and Kitwood's argument that individuals with dementia still are persons (Kitwood, 1997), to studies of language and interaction in the 1990s (Hamilton, 1994; Ramanathan, 1997), to the more recent work of Sabat (2001) and others.

A focus on storytelling as a joint activity implies a focus on its organization and performance, rather than on the individual and his or her behavior. Such an approach could most certainly be beneficial for studies of the persons with dementia in interaction with other persons. In particular, it allows an understanding of how the participants jointly deal with the consequences of cognitive and linguistic loss. Starting with storytelling as a joint activity thus implies that it is not the individual with dementia who is the prime focus but rather the activities involving persons in the everyday network and the way these persons jointly take on the problems caused by the progressing disease (Hydén, 2014).

One of the basic tenets of joint activities is *collaboration*: the participants must *coordinate* their storytelling actions and listening in such a way that all the participants can construct roughly the same story. This collaboration presupposes that all the participants monitor each other and themselves so mutual meaning making becomes possible. This can be done in three steps:

1   The teller must design (or construct) story utterances for the listeners, that is, tell the story in such a way that the teller can expect the listener to understand the story.

2   The listeners must listen to and interpret utterances as if they are designed for them to understand, that is, as if they are meaningful and fit into the emerging story.

3   Together, all participants must mutually check their interpretations of the utterances so they construct roughly the same story – otherwise the storytelling will result in confusion, because the participants will discuss widely different stories although they aim at talking about the same story.

In order for this mutual *meaning-making process* to work, a storyteller never tells a whole story in one long sequence. Rather, the story is partitioned into smaller parts, each part roughly corresponding to an 'idea unit' (Gee, 1986). This could be conceptualised in interactional terms as the teller making *contributions* to the ongoing storytelling activity – and each contribution corresponds to an idea. Each contribution is marked by a small pause – often less than half a second long, giving the participants a possibility to signal their understanding or request a clarification. From a cognitive perspective this makes it easier for the participants to understand and construct the emerging story, and from an interactional perspective it becomes possible to check for mutual understanding.

How stories are sectioned into smaller units can be seen in Example 1. It is an extract from a joint interview with a woman and her husband about their life both before and after the dementia diagnosis. Both are around 70 years old and have been married for more than 40 years. The wife, Ann, received an Alzheimer's disease diagnosis seven years before the first interview, while her husband Carl is healthy. Ann has profound problems identifying events and sometimes also constructing utterances. The couple is part of a longitudinal project based on annual joint interviews with couples with dementia. This couple has been interviewed three times, and Example 1 is from the second interview. Just before the start of the extracted part of the interview, the interviewer had asked the couple if they could tell about what has happened during the year since the previous interview. Ann starts to tell about her everyday life.

Example 1.

```
1   Ann: yes it obviously happens very much due to my
         alzheimer (0.4)
2        .hh 'cause it goes like this ((hand movements
         up and down))
3        but right now it has levelled out ((illustrates
         with hand movement)) (0.5)
4        eh and this affects you eh (0.3)
5        'cause I have temperament now so .hh (0.4)
6        and I can (0.5) become sad sometimes and (0.7)
7        eh and I cannot not understand why I become like
         this
```

Although Ann can construct longer units of talk, they are sometimes not 'correct' grammatically or she cannot find a word or an expression (Lines 2 and 3) and sometimes uses a gesture in a possible attempt to substitute for the word or expression (Lines 2 and 3). When Ann tells about her everyday life, she tells about how her 'alzheimer' affects her life – and how difficult it is for her to understand what is happening to her. She tells her story by introducing one 'idea' or 'theme' at a time. The first idea is the fact that she is affected by her 'alzheimer' (Line 1). This is followed by a pause (0.4 seconds). The second idea is that her disease goes up and down (Line 2). She continues by introducing new ideas, every time ending with pauses. In the pauses, her husband and the two interviewers have the potential to raise questions or request a repetition – which none of them do. Instead they continue to look at her and in that way signal that they are active listeners waiting for her next contribution.

Ann continues her story. In Example 2, from a part of the interview almost immediately after the end of Example 1, she tries to be more specific about the challenges she faces and the fact that she becomes quite angry when she cannot follow an ongoing conversation with her husband. The structure is the same as in Example 1: small contributions followed by pauses.

Example 2.

```
1   Ann:  I know (0.6)
2         but (0.9)
3         there is not much you can (1.0)
4         still it is is (1.3)
5         it's when I think I cannot do things I get
          angry and so .hh (0.8)
6         so then I notice (.) things happen
7   Carl:((looks at his wife)) a: you are sad about the
         illness=
```

```
8   Ann:   =yes((looks at her husband))
9   Carl:  because you have problems with listening when
           we talk .hh
```

In Example 2 there are not only pauses surrounding each contribution but also a number of hesitations marked by longer pauses, often longer than in Example 1. It is as if Ann is searching for words and expressions and cannot find them (Lines 2–4). It is not until Line 5 that Ann finds the words that can express her feelings, although she has difficulty finishing her next utterance (Line 6). Carl steps in and offers an interpretation by saying that Ann is sad about the illness (Line 7) – something Ann immediately supports (Line 8).

Example 2 adds a new aspect of collaboration when Carl adds contributions to the story. As a result, the story at first told by Ann turns into a shared story told by both Ann and Carl. The story is told collaboratively through a number of small steps – contributions – when the participants add new elements to the story. Each contribution has to be noted and understood by the other participant, otherwise some kind of repair becomes necessary until both participants can accept the (negotiated) meaning of the contribution. Storytelling is thus collaboration in which participants together tell, interpret and construct a shared story.

Common ground

Storytelling as a collaborative activity – as conversations in general – has its own economy. One basic economic principle is, never say more than is needed (Grice, 1975). One reason for this principle is that it makes storytelling – and conversations in general – easier and quicker. The teller, for instance, just needs to introduce a new character once and then use personal pronouns to refer to that character again; or, if the participants know each other well, few explanations are needed when a specific event or person is mentioned because the teller can safely assume that the other already is familiar with the reference. Further, this economic principle becomes even more prominent when people tell *shared stories* (Lerner, 1992). These are stories about events and experiences that they both shared: both have first-hand knowledge about the subject matter and both of them are likely to have told and heard the story before. Shared stories imply equal epistemic status and rights, that is, both participants 'know' what happened and hence have the right to judge the story told, whether or not it is true (Heritage, 2012). Telling shared stories is common especially if the participants have known each other over a long period of time, something that is common for spouses who have been married for a long time, longtime friends or people who have worked together for many years.

The shared knowledge a couple has established between themselves during their relationship constitutes what often is called their *common ground* (Clark, 1996). From a social–psychological perspective, common ground is not a set of specific knowledge but is rather about the spouses' *mutual assumptions and expectations*. The first spouse can safely assume and expect that the second spouse is familiar with certain salient references (e.g. date of marriage, name of grandchildren, first time they met, what they usually do on Saturday nights, etc.). The first spouse can also assume and expect that the second spouse assumes and expects the same of the first spouse, that is, that she knows about Saturday nights, etc. The same is of course true for the second spouse: she, too, assumes that the first spouse knows about Saturday nights, and so on. Basically there is no end to this spiral of mutual assumptions and expectations (Clark, 1996). Following Clark, common ground is concerned with shared biographical knowledge and shared situational knowledge. The storyteller can further assume a third kind of common ground, namely their shared general cultural and social knowledge: London is a city, Shakespeare lived before Milton, Manchester United plays football, etc. (Clark, 1996).

Having a common ground, one spouse can tell a story about the first time the couple met, that is, something she can assume and expect to belong to their common ground, and expect the other spouse to (either tacitly or explicitly) acknowledge the correctness of the assumption. Example 3 illustrates this process.

Example 3.

```
1    Carl:  eh it was at the Grouse as it was called then
2           on the main square (.)
3           a dance place (.)
4           we met there the first time
5    Ann:   [a:] we met there
```

One of the interviewers asked the spouses to tell about the first time they met. Carl starts by telling about them meeting at a dance restaurant ('the Grouse'). In doing this he addresses the interviewers but tells about something that he would expect and assume that Ann is familiar with. So his explanations about 'the Grouse' – that its name has changed and where it was located – is directed to the interviewers rather than to Ann. When Carl finishes the theme 'where we met the first time' (on Line 4), Ann immediately affirms his story (Line 5). Thus, so far in the example there is no indication of either of the spouses failing in their mutual expectations and assumptions about the other.

Common ground not only is relevant for people's shared biographies but also is central in joint activities, such as when people tell stories together. In order to be 'economic' each new utterance in the storytelling event is added to the participants' situationally emerging common ground. So by adding contributions to their common ground the participants make a stepwise progression: together they 'know' what already has transpired among them, what parts of the story already have been told, and what has happened in the story world so far (Clark, 1994; Herman, 1999). This makes it possible for the participants to constantly and jointly monitor and revise their activity and jointly construct (for all practical purposes) roughly the same story.

Fragmentation and redefinition of the common ground

Common ground depends on the participants being able to remember and 'retrieve' general, biographical and situational knowledge. This is what becomes a challenge for the person with Alzheimer's disease, as one of its primary symptoms is problems with episodic and working memory and later semantic memory (Morris & Becker, 2004). This will have profound effects on couples living with dementia as one spouse increasingly is challenged in using common ground, both in terms of being able to remember and also in terms of what to expect specifically from the other spouse. Thus, as the Alzheimer's disease progresses, the common ground of the couple slowly becomes fragmented, leaving one spouse as the prime carer of the shared past and its memories.

Spouses in all relationships from time to time face troubles in keeping up their common ground due to changing social and economic circumstances, aging and so on. The problems facing couples with dementia is that in everyday interaction the changes brought on by the dementia are manifested in the fact that the spouses' common ground starts to fragment as the person with dementia has increasing problems understanding what the healthy spouse refers to. Remembering shared past events and shared knowledge important in storytelling (names of children, date of marriage, etc.) becomes challenged. As a result, which assumptions to make and what to expect become less evident and as a consequence it becomes more difficult to use the common ground as a resource when the spouses tell stories about themselves. Further, the person with dementia will also have increasing problems with using the situational common ground, that is, remembering what has been said previously in the ongoing conversation. Finally, the person with dementia will also be challenged in referring to the social and cultural common ground, as it will be increasingly difficult for him or her to recognize generally known persons, dates and places.

The challenges around common ground are recurrent and do not go away but instead will gradually increase as times goes by. Eventually, the person with dementia will be able to recognize very few shared events and memories. As already argued, all storytellers can for different reasons have problems with their common ground, from mistakes and misunderstanding, to forgetfulness. Normally participants find and use 'local' ways to deal with these problems: clarifying, adding more information, reminding someone, negotiating experiences and 'memories', etc. What is characteristic for couples living with dementia, as well as for nurses having a professional relation to persons with dementia, is that the problems connected to an eroding common ground are *pervasive* because all kinds of interactions are affected, the problems *increase* over time and they have *profound effects* on storytelling as well as relations and identities (Hydén & Kristiansson, 2017).

Fragmentation of the couple's common ground has consequences both for storytelling activities and for the spouses' relation and their shared identity as a couple, the 'we' (Hydén & Nilsson, 2015). The reason for this is that common ground is not only about cognitive and communicative expectations but also about *relational* and *moral assumptions and expectations*. It is as if the healthy spouse is saying, 'if we have this kind of relation, then I expect you to know and remember, otherwise I must reconsider our relation and who I am' (Hellström et al., 2005, 2007). This stresses the fact that most relations and identities are *interdependent* – especially when people have lived together for a long time. Thus, the eroding common ground has wide consequences besides the communicative ones.

As a consequence, the changing common ground may threaten the ongoing activity and especially the face of the person with dementia, and thus the status of the person with dementia and the interdependent relation. This development is nicely illustrated by Ann and Carl when they describe their pervasive everyday problems in making conversation (Example 4).

Example 4.

```
1    Ann:   I know (0.6)
2           but (0.9)
3           there is not much you can (1.0)
4           still it is is (1.3)
5           it's when I think I cannot do things I get
            angry and so .hh (0.8)
6           so then I notice (.) things happen
7    Carl:  ((looks at his wife)) a: you are sad about the
            illness=
8    Ann:   =yes((looks at her husband))
9    Carl:  because you have problems with listening when
            we talk .hh
10          so words ca jump away so they get lost ((looks
            at his wife))
11          and when you want to say something then she
            just has one thing in her head =
```

```
12  Ann:        a:
13  Carl:       =.hh but something quite different comes
                out of the mouth
14  Ann:        yes:
15  Carl:       =that's the reason I can give a totally
                crazy answer she thinks then
16  Ann:        ((laughs))  a:  noo  =I  just  scream
                lobotomized  ((laughs)))]
```

Ann and Carl's story is about what happens as well as an illustration of the communicative problems they have. Basically the story is about Ann's growing anger over her problems with finding words and remembering events as well as saying something that she did not intend to do. In particular, the story points out that conflicts between them emerge as a result of communicative problems (Line 15). The story is told jointly by Ann and Carl: she is presenting the theme and basic outline of the story, while Carl is supporting with phrases and interpretations when the words fail Ann – something we will return to.

Ann and Carl's situation is widely supported by researchers, who have found that one of the most painful and difficult parts of dementia for couples are the communicative problems that are a consequence of the dementia (see e.g. Small et al., 2003). Thus, learning how to deal with the eroding common ground is important.

Collaborative compensatory adaptions

One way to avoid these threats is for the spouses to find ways to deal with the changing common ground. Most of these ways are intended to compensate for what they no longer can do without effort and are often called compensatory adaptions, that is, attempts to solve, by changing something, the problems and threats posed. Compensatory adaptions are often thought of as individual strategies, but they can also involve several persons working together (Berg & Upchurch, 2007; Berg et al., 1998). These compensatory adaptions are collaborative: it is not just a question of the person with dementia changing but all participants jointly adapting to the new situation that emerges through the effect of the dementia. The collaborative compensatory adaptions cannot be just momentary, but must (1) function in many different situations, (2) be preventive in order to avoid threatening situations, and (3) be such that they can be used by all participants without a complex learning process. One simple way for spouses is to use strategies they are already familiar with because they have used them before in different situations. Most persons are accustomed to interacting in asymmetric situations, for instance when one person knows much more than the other (e.g. expert–novice; adult–child). Experiences from these kind of interactional situations may serve as a template for interaction in joint activities involving persons with dementia.

A common denominator in many of these experiences has to do with organizing the interaction between the participants in such a way that the 'expert' may support and help the 'novice' in order for the 'novice' to solve the problem by himself or herself next time. The 'expert' does this by constructing a metaphorical *scaffold*. This can be accomplished by arranging tasks, support and feedback in such a way that the 'novice' is able to solve the problem on his or her own. This has been called *scaffolding*:

> 'Scaffolding' is a process that enables the child or novice to solve a problem, carry out a task or achieve a goal which would be beyond his unassisted efforts. This scaffolding consists essentially of the adult 'controlling' those elements of the task that are initially beyond the learner's capacity, thus permitting him to concentrate upon and complete only those elements that are within his range of competence. (Wood et al., 1976, p. 90)

Most people have experience of and are familiar with scaffolding and can thus easily adopt already known interactional formats for interaction with persons with dementia – and the person with dementia can use the same familiarity in order to use the 'scaffolds'. In the following two sections, different forms of collaborative compensatory adaptions in storytelling that both involve scaffolding will be discussed: first, proactive strategies and second, strategies for joint meaning making.

Being proactive

One of the most important kinds of collaborative compensatory adaption is scaffolding and the conversational partner's help to *frame, reframe and remind* about the joint activity. One way to deal with some of the collaborative problems is for the person without dementia to be *proactive* by organising the interaction beforehand in such a way that the risk for certain problems to emerge is minimised. This means thinking ahead: first, being at least one step ahead of the next turns in the interaction; second, imagining and predicting what will happen if nothing is done; third, predicting the possible problems that may emerge; and fourth, finding alternatives like changing aspects of the situation as well as projecting (possible) alternative turns.

Being proactive in this way may involve things like changing certain aspects of the physical and social situation by, for instance, reducing distraction from other stimuli in the environment, in order to enlist the attention of the person with dementia and help him or her to keep it focused on the joint activity.

It could also mean adapting the general pace of the talk, allowing more time for the turn taking as well as other measures that increase the probability for successful participation (Müller & Guendouzi, 2005).

Being proactive might also imply suggesting and using *formats* that both the person with dementia and the other participants can use productively, that is, formats that allow for the person with dementia to participate actively and that are not face threatening. In this way disengagement and withdrawal are avoided. One way to do this is by projecting formats for next turns that are possible for the person with dementia to use and hence to continue to participate in the activity. Many persons with dementia, especially in the later stages, will provide only minimal responses or turns (Hamilton, 1994). One way to deal with this situation could of course be for the healthy person to talk more and in that way minimise the need for contributions by the person with dementia. Another, more proactive way, would be to project a possible format of the next turn, for instance by asking an open-ended question that would give the next speaker the opportunity to answer by telling a story, something that could be difficult for some persons with dementia. The opposite would be to use a closed question that just allows for a simple yes or no or some other specific information, often easier to grasp for a person with more advanced dementia (Mikesell, 2009).

One further possibility to be proactive is to tell stories that already are familiar and use a format for the telling that will be supportive so the person with dementia can continue as a participant. The telling of autobiographical stories is often based on previous tellings rather than on memories of the 'original' events. Persons with dementia quite frequently repeat the same story or story fragment over and over and it is easy to think that these fragments and repetitions are meaningless, often because it is challenging for others to listen, and to think that repetition is connected to a loss of temporal abilities (remembering that the story has already been told). Although these explanations might carry some truth, it is true that people with dementia may repeat story segments 'that capture, albeit in frozen ways, the teller's attempt at making sense of his or her life', as Ramanathan (1997, p. 115) once wrote. In line with this argument, it is thus possible to regard repetitions as a form of reuse of already existing story elements, from the abstract story structure, to specific 'sentences' and verbal expressions, to phonological units like words. In fact, most speakers use already used linguistic elements in new situations and linguistic contexts because it makes speaking quicker and easier as new forms do not need to be constructed just then.

As a consequence, using already used and established forms and units might be an important help for persons with dementia as they face word-finding and memory difficulties. Thus, repetitions can be regarded as a creative use of already established narrative and linguistic elements in order to solve interactional and communicative challenges. So suggesting and using well-established stories might be a good strategy – although at the same time it implies a risk because of the changing and fragmented common ground, as can be seen in Example 5 from the opening of the first interview with Ann and Carl. One of the interviewers has asked the couple whether they could tell about the first time they met. Ann quickly hands over the responsibility for the telling to Carl.

Example 5.

```
1    Ann:  you start ((laughs and puts her hand on her
           forehead))
2    Carl: well:: it was nineteen sixty-eight (2.0)
3          so it was (.)
4          in January
5    Ann:  a: yes it was .hh a
6    Carl: eh it was at the Grouse as it was called then
7          on the main square (.)
8          a dance place (.)
9          we met there the first time
10   Ann:  [a:] we met there
11   Carl: yes then after that
12   Ann:  .hh yeah
13   Carl: we have kept together of course
14   Ann:  .hh yeah
15   Carl: we got engaged (2.0) do you remember?
16   Ann:  eh. no ((laughs))
17   Carl: no ((laughs))
18   Ann:  ((laughs)) have not remembered that too far
           away I think
19   Carl: no. seventy
20         then seventy-one we married
```

Ann and Carl have probably told this story many times, both for others but also between themselves. It is a story about an important moment in their relationship, the first time they met and the consequences of this encounter. Thus it involves a number of shared memories about places and dates. The mutual assumptions and expectations around this story are of course important because they concern events that defined and still define Ann and Carl as a couple. Not remembering these events or parts of the story can be expected to be something that is charged with emotional meaning. Maybe Ann's quick handing over of the telling to Carl can be seen as a way to preemptively deal with the risk of not being able to tell the story. Some evidence for this interpretation can be found in her gesture: she puts her hand on her forehead as if she has problems remembering. But as she performs this gesture she concurrently laughs as if minimising the value of her gesture. And maybe Carl senses Ann's hesitancy as he quickly starts to tell the story.

When Carl starts to tell the story, Ann is signaling a state of attention: she is sitting erect, listening. Carl starts by giving the year for their first encounter (Line 2) and then adds it was in January – something Ann affirms (Line 5). The fact that Ann chooses to explicitly confirm the month rather than year might have to do with a possible evaluation of the year as easier to remember while the month is a bit more difficult. Thus, confirming the month might be seen by the interviewers and Carl as an indication that Ann actually shares the couple's common ground. In other words, it is a way for Ann to secure her face against the threat of losing memories.

As Carl continues, Ann confirms the place (Line 10) and Carl's evaluation of the story: 'after that we have kept together of course' (Lines 11–14). But then Carl adds something new: a question directed at Ann about what year they got engaged. This type of question is often found among couples with dementia (Small & Perry, 2005) and has been called 'questions with known answers' by Ekström and Majlesi (2017). It is a question that puts Ann in an awkward position: she must find the correct answer; otherwise she might come across as a less capable person. She quickly admits that she cannot remember the year and adds that she actually has not forgotten but she has chosen not to remember because it is 'too far away' (Line 18). Carl then supplies the year.

So telling this story was safe because they had most probably told the story before. At the same time, it involved risks of indications of forgetfulness that could be face threatening to Ann. The collaborative compensatory strategies they used were based on a division of work: Carl tells the story and Ann affirms Carl's contributions, which makes it possible for Ann to actually continue as an active participant in the telling about the salient event. This works until Carl asks her about a specific date, something Ann cannot provide. Thus this example shows both the possibilities of scaffolding by telling a known story and also the potential problems with breaking away from the scaffolding format and instead introducing what could be called a 'teaching' format: asking questions with known answers.

Joint meaning making and repair

As many of the examples have indicated, the changes of the common ground result in a challenge for the participant in their joint meaning making: something is not there because the person with dementia cannot find either a word or phrase or a referent (a specific fact, event or date) – or both. The challenges connected to joint meaning making will increase as the dementia progresses; at a later phase of the dementia, the person will make very few if any active contributions to the conversation or storytelling (Hamilton, 1994). Although this is the case, research shows that both the person with dementia and their healthy partner have a strong motivation and inclination to continue talking together and telling stories and thus to engage in collaborative compensatory work. This might imply that the participants actively strive to *repair* whatever meaning-making problems they face. These repairs often become extended and involve the active participation of all parties. It will also become clear that many of the challenges the spouses face have to do with the changing common ground, and these changes will also have consequences for the repair work they must engage in.

Central to extended, collaborative repair is its aim to *increase the likelihood for establishing joint meaning*. This implies that extended, collaborative repair work involves the participants' creative abilities: they have to set up the problem (the joint understanding) in such a way that it is solvable for them, allowing them to find solutions by using various semiotic resources (words, nonverbal vocalization, gestures, etc.).

Example 6 is from the second interview with Ann and Carl. Ann's memory challenges have become quite pronounced and she often cannot find names, places or dates. The example is from the beginning of the interview, and she tells about her life with Alzheimer's disease (it is a continuation of Examples 1, 2 and 4).

Example 6.

```
1    Ann:   but all this is part of the alzheimers .hh you
            walk around during the night (0.6)
2           once upon a time .hh
3           I used to work at a nursing home or ((looks at
            her husband))
4           well something [like that]
5    Carl:              [yes at] St George's °I think it was°
6    Ann:   and I did learn a lot (0.5) =
7           I had a (.) small lady that I loved (0.2)
            ((laughs)) (.)
8           and she walked around through the nights back
            and forth .hh
9           with a cup of coffe which she turned like this
            ((demonstrates how coffee is poured out)) into
            the flower vase (.)
```

When Ann is telling about her own walking around at night, she is reminded of a lady she met when she worked as a nurse at a nursing home for people with dementia (Lines 2 and 3) and she wants to tell about this lady. She starts by introducing a small story abstract (Line 3), but in doing so she cannot find the name of the nursing home. She indicates her trouble already in the linguistic construct when she says she 'used to work at a nursing home', then she adds the word 'or'. This word might (at least in Swedish) indicate that the teller is unsure about something. The small word 'or' might be seen as an attempt to self-repair – or at least an indication of trouble. Ann also directs her gaze at her husband. In the interviews with the couples with dementia, one of the most used devices for signaling a need for support and help is turning the gaze towards the healthy spouse. Ann directs her gaze towards her husband but probably finds him slow in responding so she says, 'well something like that'. Ann often uses this kind of face work in the interviews: she 'brushes' away face-threatening situations by degrading the social value of the knowledge she cannot remember. She did the same in Example 5 above when she could not remember the engagement date. Simultaneously as Ann is saying that it does not matter, Carl starts to support her with the information she requested: she worked at a nursing home called St George's. Ann accepts this information and continues her story.

At the end of her story Ann once more has troubles finding a phrase (Line 9). She obviously cognitively 'knows' what to say, but she cannot find words and a construction that fits. As in the previous repair case (Line 3) Ann first attempts to self-repair. In that case she could not find a way to repair her indicated trouble and Carl eventually provided the name. In this case Ann uses a gesture for the phrase she cannot find: she enacts pouring the contents of a coffee cup. Directly after the gestures she adds information about the coffee being poured into a flower vase. In other words, Ann could not find the linguistic part of her utterance having to do with pouring a cup (the verb construction), although the rest of the utterance worked.

Example 6 thus illustrates (1) how troubles are noticed and signaled, (2) the preference for self-repair on the part of the person with dementia, and (3) how when that does not work the healthy spouse can support information. In supporting Ann, Carl is making use of the couple's common ground: both Ann and Carl potentially know the name of the nursing home.

In the third interview with Ann and Carl, Ann's memory problems have become quite severe. At this point in time Ann spends five days a week at a center for daily activities. She arrives around nine in the morning, and Carl comes and gets her around three in the afternoon. Ann basically cannot remember recent events and has severe problems with remembering long-ago events. In Example 7, one of the interviewers has asked Ann to describe an ordinary day at the day center. As Ann at first cannot find anything to say (not in the example), Carl starts by suggesting that Ann sings while at the center (Line 1).

Example 7.

```
1    Carl:  you often sing don't you
2    Ann:   yes sure
3    Carl:  and then you dance
4    Ann:   yes that's true
5    Carl:  and you
6    Ann:   I must tell you
7           although I'm sitting here and don't remember
            things
8           I'm very (0.5)
9           curious about what comes
10   Carl:  mm
11          what did you say
12   Ann:   I'm saying
13          I'm very curious about when I come
14          because I don't have to call and ask
15   Carl:  No
16   Ann:   No
17          then I can do something about it
18          then you come
19   Carl:  Yes
20          and then you do trips
21          and storytelling
22   Ann:   Yes
```

The fact that Carl takes the initiative can be seen as part of a repair: Ann wanted to respond to the question but cannot find anything; she sits still looking in front of her as if searching for something. She does not attempt to initiate a self-repair nor does she look at Carl for support. As Carl does spend some time at the day center where Ann spends her days, he shares at least potentially some common ground with Ann about what goes on at the center. It is also obvious that Ann cannot use her own memories nor their common ground in order to answer the interviewer's question. So when Carl suggests that Ann sings, he is vicariously invoking the couple's common ground: he is providing some information pertaining to the common ground that Ann cannot. Carl is putting forward the notion of singing activities as a suggestion: 'you often sing don't you'. Suggesting makes it possible for Ann to use this utterance, by treating it as a question to which she gives an affirmative answer (Line 2).

One possibility for Ann at this point would be to continue telling about her days by adding new examples of activities. But she stops after her affirmation. Instead Carl adds a new suggestion – from their potential common ground – this time, dancing (Line 3). Again Ann confirms that she dances but does not add new items, and Carl starts to suggest a new activity (Line 5). This time Ann takes the word before Carl finishes and reflexively turns on the situation: she comments that she cannot 'remember things' (Line 7). Her next contributions (Lines 8 and 9) are quite difficult to understand. One possibility is that Ann is starting on one contribution on Line 8 – 'I'm very' – but she does not complete it, and then forgets what she wanted to say, something that is supported by the brief pause. Instead she continues in a new direction, saying 'curious about what comes'. Carl indicates that he does not understand and asks her what she means (Line 11). Then Ann makes a repair by saying that she wonders when she comes and that she does not have to call for him. She might be referring to when Carl comes and gets her in the afternoon and that she does not have to call for him. Carl does not request any more information but moves on to suggest another activity they have at the center, going on trips and telling stories (Lines 20 and 21) – something Ann confirms.

This example illustrates how both Ann and Carl try to establish joint meaning making and keep Ann in the conversation. It is noticeable that Ann's contributions are becoming smaller and that Carl takes over much of the responsibility for the storytelling, like introducing themes, suggesting elaborations, etc. In pursuing the conversation Carl primarily refers to the common ground, although Ann has severe problems remembering events. What is very clear in the example is the fact that the problems become substantial not only when Carl and Ann are talking about something shared but even more complicated when they try to use their common ground for repairing: they basically also need to repair the repair attempts.

Summary and discussion

People living with dementia not only can tell stories and participate in storytelling – they actually do it most of the time. Over time – as Alzheimer's disease progresses – the person with dementia will become increasingly challenged both in telling stories and taking part in storytelling events. As this chapter demonstrated, it is possible to sustain the active participation of the person through the establishment of collaborative relations with other, healthy participants who can support and facilitate the joint storytelling. A main strategy the participant can use is scaffolding, that is, re-organizing the responsibilities in the storytelling activity in order to facilitate for the person with dementia.

It is at the same time obvious that persons living with dementia face increasing challenges as storytellers as the disease progresses – something not discussed in this chapter. These challenges will affect their possibilities to participate but also to present their own voice, that is, their specific, individual biographical perspective on events and in constructing the story. Over time it is instead the other participants who will tell the stories and thus give voice to the specific perspectives of the person with dementia. Thus, in the stories told in the later stages of dementia the *vicarious voices* of the healthy storyteller will be stronger (Hydén, 2008). It will increasingly be the task of the healthy storyteller to hold the person with dementia as a unique individual with a specific identity and biography (Lindemann, 2014).

References

Berg, C. A., Meegan, S. P. & Deviney, F. P. (1998). A social-contextual model of coping with everyday problems across the lifespan. *International Journal of Behavioral Development, 22*, 239–261.

Berg, C. A. & Upchurch, R. (2007). A developmental-contextual model of couples coping with chronic illness across the adult life span. *Psychological Bulletin, 133*, 920–954.

Clark, H. H. (1994). Discourse in production. In M. A. Gernsbacher (Ed.), *Handbook of Psycholinguistics* (pp. 985–1021). San Diego: Academic Press.

Clark, H. H. (1996). *Using Language*. New York: Cambridge University Press.

Ekström, A. & Majlesi, A. R. (2017). Questions with known answers in interaction with people with dementia.

Gee, J. P. (1986). Units in the production of narrative discourse. *Discourse Processes, 9*, 391–422.

Grice, P. (1975). Logic and conversation. In P. Cole & J. Morgan (Eds.), *Syntax and Semantics, Vol 3: Speech Acts* (pp. 41–58). New York: Academic Press.

Gubrium, J. F. (1986). The social preservation of mind: The Alzheimer's disease experience. *Symbolic Interaction, 9*, 37–51.

Hamilton, H. E. (1994). *Conversations with an Alzheimer's Patient: An Interactional Sociolinguistic Study*. New York: Cambridge University Press.

Hellström, I., Nolan, M. & Lundh, U. (2005). We do things together: A case study of couplehood in dementia. *Dementia, 4*, 7–22.

Hellström, I., Nolan, M. & Lundh, U. (2007). Sustaining 'couplehood': Spouses' strategies for living positively with dementia. *Dementia, 6*, 383–409.

Heritage, J. (2012). The epistemic engine: Sequence organization and territories of knowledge. *Research on Language and Social Interaction, 45*, 30–52.

Herman, D. (Ed.). (1999). *Narratologies: New Perspectives on Narrative Analysis*. Columbus, OH: Ohio State University Press.

Hydén, L. C. (2008). Broken and vicarious voices in narratives. In L. C. Hydén & J. Brockmeier (Eds.), *Health, Culture and Illness: Broken Narratives* (pp. 36–53). New York: Routledge.

Hydén, L. C. (2014). How to do things with others: Joint activities involving persons with Alzheimer's disease. In L. C. Hydén, H. Lindemann & J. Brockmeier (Eds.), *Beyond Loss: Dementia, Identity, and Personhood* (pp. 137–154). New York: Oxford University Press.

Hydén, L. C. (2017). *Entangled Narratives: Collaborative Storytelling and the Re-Imagining of Dementia*. New York: Oxford University Press.

Hydén, L. C. & Kristiansson, M. (2017). Collaborative remembering in dementia: The perspective from activity theory. In M. Meade, A. J. Barnier, P. Van Bergen, C. B. Harris & J. Sutton (Eds.), *Collaborative Remembering: How Remembering with Others Influences Memory*. New York: Oxford University Press.

Hydén, L. C. & Nilsson, E. (2015). Couples with dementia: Positioning the 'we'. *Dementia, 14,* 716–733.

Kellas, J. K. (2005). Family ties: Communicating identity through jointly told family stories. *Communication Monographs, 72,* 365–389.

Kitwood, T. (1997). *Dementia Reconsidered: The Person Comes First.* Philadelphia: Open University Press.

Lerner, G. H. (1992). Assisted storytelling: Deploying shared knowledge as a practical matter. *Qualitative Sociology, 15,* 247–271.

Lindemann, H. (2014). *Holding and Letting Go: The Social Practice of Personal Identities.* New York: Oxford University Press.

Mandelbaum, J. (1987). Couples sharing stories. *Communication Quarterly, 35* (Spring), 144–171.

McKeown, J., Clarke, A. & Repper, J. (2006). Life story work in health and social care: Systematic literature review. *Journal of Advanced Nursing, 55,* 237–247.

Mikesell, L. (2009). Conversational practices of a frontotemporal dementia patient and his interlocutors. *Research on Language and Social Interaction, 42,* 135–162.

Morris, R. & Becker, J. (Eds.). (2004). *Cognitive Neuropsychology of Alzheimer's Disease* (2nd ed.). Oxford: Oxford University Press.

Müller, N. & Guendouzi, J. A. (2005). Order and disorder in conversation: Encounters with dementia of the Alzheimers type. *Clinical Linguistics and Phonetics, 19,* 393–404.

Ramanathan, V. (1997). *Alzheimer Discourse: Some Sociolinguistic Dimensions.* Mahwah, NJ: Lawrence Erlbaum Associates.

Sabat, S. R. (2001). *Experience of Alzheimer's Disease: Life Through a Tangled Veil.* Oxford: Blackwell.

Small, J. A., Gutman, G. & Hillhouse, S. M. B. (2003). Effectiveness of communication strategies used by caregivers of persons with Alzheimers disease during activities of daily living. *Journal of Speech, Language and Hearing Research, 46,* 353–367.

Small, J. A. & Perry, J. (2005). Do you remember? How caregivers question their spouses who have Alzheimers disease and the impact on communication. *Journal of Speech, Language and Hearing Research, 48,* 125–136.

Wood, D., Bruner, J. & Ross, G. (1976). The role of tutoring in problem solving. *Journal of Child Psychology and Psychiatry, 17,* 89–100.

8

DEMENTIA AS CHRONIC ILLNESS: MAINTAINING INVOLVEMENT IN EVERYDAY LIFE

Ingrid Hellström and Annika Taghizadeh Larsson

Introduction

This chapter aims at discussing the significance of relations and support from other people in order for people with dementia to sustain a sense of agency and self throughout the process of the disease departing from an understanding of dementia as a *chronic illness*. In short, this means that we will focus on the meaning of dementia, the social organisation of the world of the persons in question and the strategies used in adaptation (Conrad, 1987). While there has been a growing interest in these issues during recent decades among scholars from various disciplines, not least sociology (e.g. Gubrium, 1987), approaching dementia as a chronic illness in this sense could still be considered as a novel approach. In the chapter we will apply a conceptual framework originally developed by Corbin and Strauss (1985), focusing on how people with chronic conditions and their spouses manage serious illness at home in the context of their personal lives.

Corbin and Strauss (1985) identified three differing lines of *work* in which people with chronic illness and their spouses engage over time: *illness-related work*, *everyday work* and *biographical work*. Considerable importance was attached to biographical work, which are people's efforts to redefine and reintegrate their biographical identity in the face of chronic illness.

While Corbin and Strauss's framework has been extensively cited and used (e.g. Boeije et al., 2002; Ville, 2005; Williams, 2000), its applicability in the context of dementia, as well as in old age, remains largely unexplored.

In the chapter we will turn our attention to the everyday life at home of people living with dementia, their next-of-kin and formal caregivers, especially how the person living with dementia maintains involvement (Keady, 1999) during the course of the disease by a variety of strategies and types of work. By applying the theoretical framework suggested by Corbin and Strauss, we will highlight that people with dementia, their spouses and their carers actually have to *do* a lot of work in order manage the illness trajectory. The goal is to better understand life with dementia and what this implies for the people involved, as well as the impact of different care systems in shaping everyday life with dementia.

Dementia – a chronic illness

First, we need to deliberate what dementia is:

> Dementia is a syndrome which may be caused by a number of illnesses. The main features are of progressive decline in all aspects of cerebral function. (Jacques, 1988, p. 1)

Like other chronic diseases, such as diabetes and multiple sclerosis among others, dementia is 'long term, uncertain, expensive, often multiple, disproportionately intrusive, and [it requires] palliation' (Strauss et al., 1984, p. 16).

After a person with probable dementia has received the diagnosis, he or she embarks on a journey which is often referred to as *the illness trajectory*. To date, dementia diseases are not possible to cure, and the illness trajectory lasts several years, *it is long term* and it is not always possible to define the exact onset of the disease. With regard to this trajectory, Gubrium (1987) argues that the discourse of Alzheimer's disease uses *developmental language* (1987, p. 1) to allude to the different stages associated with this illness. And this language is also used by people living with dementia and their families. This could be illustrated by a husband talking about his wife's Alzheimer's disease:

> I have read a little about it on the Internet, there is a great deal written on the subject. Among other things I have found a list describing the symptoms within one to two or one to three years and the symptoms after three to four and in the end it's only shit everything. We are still within one to three years according to this list, she has no severe symptoms of any kind that are handicapping, it is only the short-term memory. (Hellström et al., 2005, p. 283)

He is here referring to stages of the disease and what you could expect on this specific stage, or 'according to the list'. We often mention different symptoms connected to a dementia disease, with memory disturbances as the most common. It is also common to treat the syndrome of dementia, in other words the group of the large number of different dementia diagnoses and the people living with different dementia diagnoses, as a homogenous group. These different diagnoses share the feature of *uncertainty* – a *trajectory uncertainty* (Conrad, 1987, p. 8); they seldom follow 'the list' on an individual level. To look upon people living with dementia as a homogenous group, you could, probably with good intention, refrain from the medical model. However, placing the medical model and the social model in two different pools will not serve the good of people living with dementia. This could lead to a one-dimensional view within both pools. Without question, a dementia disease implies cognitive impairment and is defined within the medical model. Otherwise, we could have kept the older concept of *senility*. During the nineteenth century, an emerging nosological trend described disease entities systematically in the medical literature, for example senile dementia was for the first time defined in 1838 (Fox, 1989). Since then a large body of research has focused on the relationship between senility and, foremost, Alzheimer's disease (e.g. Newton, 1948). In 1978, a consensus was reached among researchers – Alzheimer's disease and senile dementia were unified and this unit should not be regarded as part normal aging (Ballenger, 2006).

However, old age is the most common risk factor for dementia (Lobo et al., 2000) and if we then add the feature 'often multiple' (because the prevalence of multiple concomitant chronic conditions increases with age, to 78% among people over 80 years (van den Akker et al., 1998), the result is a variety of clinical pictures and difficulties associated with the diagnosis of dementia. In addition, the dementia disease itself could 'multiple' if the person with dementia does not receive proper treatment and care for his or her different conditions. While the medical perspective on dementia may still hold a strong position, the insight that the consequences of a dementia diagnosis are not given or purely medical is not by any means new. Different conditions might lead to disabilities, for example memory problems in dementia. Around 1965 Kahn and colleagues launched the concept of *excess disabilities*, and Kahn explains:

> we called it excess disability, where the functional disability was greater than that warranted by actual physical and physiological impairment of the *individual*. (Kahn, 1965, p. 112)

Since then studies have shown that it is possible to influence the *excess disabilities* of people with dementia in different ways by tailoring the care to the individual (i.e. Brody et al., 1971; Rogers et al., 2000) – with a more modern term – in a person-centred way. The concept of *excess disabilities* has also been used in combination with Kitwood's (1997) *malignant social psychology* (Sabat, 1994), which contains a list of elements of how caregivers can harm the personhood and the well-being of the person living with dementia, that is, by labelling the person with negative metaphors – for example as a zombie (Behuniak, 2011) – or that a person with dementia label himself or herself as a vegetable, quoting a man with Alzheimer's disease:

> But, obviously it's a sad development to become a vegetable. That you don't wish for, of course. But you don't have much of a choice. (Hellström, 2009, p. 106)

Treating a person with dementia according to these types of negative metaphors could also lead to the person not receiving proper treatment and *palliation* for his or her symptoms connected to the dementia disease, for example depression or pain.

After introducing his biopsychological framework (Kitwood, 1988) in dementia research, Kitwood (1997) argued in the 1990s that adverse environmental conditions could increase the symptoms of a dementia disease and stressed the importance of supportive interpersonal relations in order to improve the situation for people living with dementia. A general understanding of dementia seems to be that people who have it run the risk of losing their identity and personhood and that it will lead to a total dependency, and 'vulnerable' and 'dependent' are words commonly used to describe persons with dementia. However, by acknowledging dementia as a chronic illness, we can see that on an individual level, persons living with a chronic disease and their families are able to adjust to symptoms and can influence how specific symptoms are experienced on a daily basis, even though they sometimes are *disproportionately intrusive* and *expensive* for the whole family, with regard to extra burden in, for example, housework and expenses connected to early retirement and medical costs. Departing from an understanding of dementia as a chronic illness also raises a need to acknowledge that the social and cultural context of life with dementia matters and that, for example, cross-cultural differences in the meaning and treatment of illness may contribute to variations in how life with dementia is experienced and manifested (c.f. Conrad, 1987).

Adjusting in everyday life

The unique person living with dementia adjusts to his or her cognitive impairment, most often in relation to other people, family members and friends. This happens even though everybody affected by the disease has a unique illness trajectory and can therefore adjust to the diagnosis in different ways. It is important to distinguish between the course of illness and the illness trajectory. The course of illness is described in biomedical terms, that is, the different stages connected to Alzheimer's disease. On the other hand, as acknowledged by Corbin and Strauss (1988), the illness trajectory is each person's unique accommodation to a chronic illness, together with their care partner, and the impact of the illness on their daily life and the work that is needed. Thus, an understanding of everyday life with a dementia disease needs to be anchored on an understanding of relatedness since intimate relationships between the person with dementia and his or her significant others or primary caregivers are instrumental to maintaining a sense of agency and self in dementia. Existing empirical work within dementia research suggests that multidimensional and dynamic interrelationships between persons with dementia and their significant others or carers occur throughout the entire experience of dementia. Researchers have explored the relational elements of caring in dementia from the perspective of the caregiver. These studies have shed some light on the interactive personal experiences involved, highlighting the fact that most carers invest considerable efforts in sustaining the self-esteem and sense of agency of the person with dementia, even if their actual contribution to the relationship diminishes over time. In most caring relationships, the main motivation throughout the entire process is to maintain the involvement of the persons being cared for by creating ways in which their sense of agency and self can be sustained for as long as possible. Adding to the more established biomedical and personhood lens within dementia research, several scholars (e.g. Bartlett & O'Connor, 2007; Boyle, 2008; Kelly & Innes, 2013; Nedlund & Nordh, 2015; Örulv, 2012; Österholm & Hydén, 2014) have during the last decade argued for the importance of taking the wider social and cultural context into account and of acknowledging people with dementia not only as patients or as persons interacting with others but also as citizens and active agents whose lives and opportunities following the onset of dementia are also shaped by welfare systems and by social structures related to gender, ethnicity, class, etc.

Thus, insights brought forward by scholars studying chronic illness could not be considered as new within dementia research. However, communication between dementia researchers focusing on the relational and social dimensions of dementia and researchers in the field of chronic illness still seems to be quite scarce. Furthermore, to date it has been rare to apply specific theoretical frames developed within research on chronic illness in the context of dementia. Consequently, important opportunities to explore and highlight differences as well as similarities between life with dementia and other chronic diseases remain.

In the following we will give some examples of how, during the illness trajectory, persons living with dementia and their care partners maintain involvement in everyday life. We use the three lines of work originally developed by Corbin and Strauss (1985) focusing on how people with chronic conditions and their spouses manage serious illness at home in the context of their personal lives. As part of this, we will illustrate how the social and cultural context may play a crucial role for how everyday life with dementia is played out. Drawing on two case studies, we will show how some people living with dementia in today's Sweden may maintain involvement in everyday life at home, also in the later stages of the disease, through relationships and varying, changing and creative forms of interaction not only with family members, but also with formal caregivers in the form of *personal assistance*.

Personal assistance and dementia

The introduction of personal assistance and the related system of direct payment represents a significant step towards 'full citizenship' for many people with disabilities in countries like the United Kingdom and Sweden in the sense that their opportunities to take control over their own living conditions were significantly improved. Ideologically, the introduction of this support system was a prominent development within disability policy and activism: that the right to live like others, including to be self-determinant and autonomous, for people with extensive disabilities can be realized through personal assistants who serve as the so-called assistance users' 'arms and legs', while the assistance users determine what should be done and how. In Sweden, a person who is granted personal assistance and so-called attendance allowance receives payment corresponding to the number of hours of assistance she or he is assessed to need and may then choose to organise the assistance by support from the municipality, a cooperative or a private company. The person can also choose to be her or his own assistance provider. However, the conditions are such that personal assistance has to be granted before the age of 65, and the amount of assistance accorded cannot be increased after the 65th birthday of the person who had the entitlement (Jönson & Taghizadeh Larsson, 2009). Thus, concerning people with dementia, only those who are in need of extensive support in their daily life before the age of 65 may be entitled to personal assistance.

The two persons with dementia who participated in the case studies both received their dementia diagnosis at a relatively young age and had extensive care needs when they reached the age of 65. One of the case studies involved a 72-year-old man ('Tage'), diagnosed with frontotemporal dementia 13 years previously, his wife and personal assistants. The other involved a woman aged 66 ('Monika'), diagnosed with Alzheimer's disease 11 years previously, her husband and personal assistants. The two case studies comprise a variety of empirical materials (participant observations inside and outside the home of the participant, video recordings and audio-recorded interviews with spouses and assistants) and seem to be the first to explore the phenomenon of living with dementia supported by personal assistants.

Illness-related work

The two persons with dementia who participated in the case studies both were at a phase in their individual illness trajectories when they no longer could use spoken language or move from one place to another without assistance. Thus, a lot of illness-related work had to be accomplished by the personal assistants and the spouses in order to meet their needs of eating, going to the toilet or changing incontinence pads, staying warm and clean, sleeping, taking medication, moving around, dealing with contacts with health-care professionals, etc. In fact – and as told by Monika's husband at a later contact – from a medical perspective Monika was considered as being at the very last stage of the disease, and of her life. Just a couple of weeks after the researcher (ATL) visited Monika and her husband, Monika's physician had a meeting with the husband aimed at preparing him for the end-of-life phase and to get the husband's views on life-sustaining treatment. According to the physician, the disease would soon inhibit vital bodily functions and lead to death. Illustrating the uncertainty of medical prognosis in people with dementia, more than a year and a half later, Monika is still living at home with her husband and personal assistants.

Apart from care work such as dressing, feeding and dental care, regular efforts were also invested in maintaining bodily functioning. Every morning, before Monika was helped out of bed with the lift, she was given massage in her bed. During the day, now and then, Monika's husband made Monika stand on her legs and slither across the floor while holding her closely under her arms and slowly taking one step at a time backwards. Similarly, referring to Tage's physician, Tage's wife stressed the importance of supporting Tage to walk, in order for him to remember how to walk. According to her, walking was also vital to prevent blood clots. She said that she was quite sure that Tage would not have still been alive without these regular walks, which were also prescribed in a notebook used by the personal assistants and Tage's spouse for communication of information regarding Tage's care. In the notebook, it was written that Tage had to be supported to walk once every hour.

Everyday work

What types of everyday work then were carried out by the personal assistants and spouses in order to help the two persons with dementia to perform the regular activities of daily living (Corbin & Strauss, 1988)?

The two case studies provide insight concerning a variety of everyday work accomplished by, in particular, the personal assistants, whose interaction with the persons with dementia was the very focus of the participants' observations. Here, two particular forms of everyday work will be highlighted: *acknowledging routines* and *interpreting bodily and facial signs* These are overarching in their character and related to *how* it was decided what a certain day would look like in large and small. Other forms of everyday work, which could simultaneously be considered as biographical work, will be presented in the next section.

Acknowledging routines obviously meant to do very much the same thing everyday and at the same time as the day before. In contrast to residential care (see e.g. Harnett, 2010), where institutional routines known to the carers already exist somewhat independently of those who receive care, these routines had been formed and articulated when personal assistants first entered the home, in this case the home of Tage and his wife. Or as Tage's wife explained during one of the interviews, beginning with a question posed by one of Tage's first assistants:

Interviewer: What are your routines here?
Wife: Tage and I never had any routines, so I had to sit down together with the assistants and agree on what routines we would have.

These routines, formulated in cooperation with the wife, probably played a particularly important role because Tage no longer could communicate in spoken language how he wanted a certain day to appear.

Another related and overarching kind of everyday work that, according to the participants' observations, was used by both Tage's and Monika's assistants, but only explicitly acknowledged by Tage's assistants during the interviews, was *interpreting bodily and facial signs and sounds, looking for signs of pleasure – or discontent*. As a result of interpretations of discontent, for example turning the body in a particular way, activities that were in process would be terminated or actions, such as change of position or visits to the toilet, would be carried out. Interpretations of pleasure – like facial expressions interpreted as smiles – were commented on as providing assurance that the person with dementia was enjoying the current activity. In the case of Monika, the assistants seemed to have been unaware of doing this kind of everyday work until the researcher explicitly commented on it. However, according to the participants' observations, Monika's assistants devoted much of their time to this kind of everyday work, judging from their almost constant focus and commenting on her facial expressions and on whether she seemed to be happy or discontent. Furthermore, a lot of focus was directed to her habit of squeezing her teeeth, which seemed to be interpreted as a sign of discontent or being tired.

It was obvious that the assistants invested a lot of energy in these interpretations, and that it was not an easy task for them to try to determine the meaning of Monika's or Tage's bodily and facial signs. For example, in the case of Tage, the assistants were at the time of the observations preoccupied with a new sound – wheezing – that had recently replaced his habit of whistling. Did the wheezing mean the same as the whistling, that Tage was content, or did it have another meaning?

Biographical work

Biographical work concerns the work done and the problems for both spouses in defining and maintaining identity and people's efforts to redefine and reintegrate their biographical identity in the face of chronic illness. In particular, Corbin and Strauss (1988, p. 255) conceptualise *accommodation* as biographical work that consists of actions aimed at achieving a sense of control and balance in life and giving life continuity and meaning despite bodily changes caused by the disease (Boeije et al., 2002).

Concerning biographical work, the relation to biography and identity was particularly evident in the everyday work described by Tage's and Monika's assistants that implied *acknowledging the previous preferences* of the person with dementia. These preferences, deriving from an earlier part of life, before Monika and Tage had – or were in need of – personal assistance, were mediated to the assistants by the spouses. Additionally, preferences that the person with dementia herself or himself had articulated to assistants in one way or other when this was still possible, were mediated by old assistants to those who had entered into the user-assistance relationship at a later point.

For example, Monika's personal assistants motivated daily trips with the adapted car to various destinations, cafés, tourist sights, etc. by explaining that according to Monika's husband, Monika had always loved going on trips with the car. Monika's case also highlights how technical advice and a flexible and personalized support system such as personal assistance may reduce *excess disabilities* to such an extent that an active and relatively independent life inside one's own home and in the local community may be an option even for people who are highly affected by a dementia disease.

Furthermore, Monika's spouse played an important role in supervising the assistants. A focus in this *supervision of formal caregivers* was to make sure that Monika was given the opportunity to live an active life, as similar as possible to her earlier life. Thus, the husband's efforts could also be conceptualised as biographical work and as a way of maintaining a sense of biographical continuity (c.f. Williams, 2000) in his spouse's, and the couple's, daily life, despite the very real and intrusive impact that the disease currently had on Monika's body and cognition. Apart from the activities already mentioned, Monika's daily life also included visiting friends and acquaintances, shopping, having coffee on the balcony, accompanying the assistants in the kitchen while cooking, watching TV, etc. On the weekends, the spouse took on the role of personal assistant and supported Monika and himself as a couple to continue to do things that they had been doing together before dementia entered their life.

As Monika has lost her ability to speak, she could not tell the researcher her preferences and whether she preferred to live this active life at – and outside – her (ordinary) home, or if she would prefer a quieter life in a residential care unit. However, her husband claimed with certainty that his wife still likes to live the way she did before she was affected by the disease – that is, an active and social life, and that, as before, she particularly enjoys excursions by car and spending time in the sun. What the researcher saw and heard during the days that she followed Monika from morning until night provided no reasons to question the spouse's assessment. In line with the daily work performed by Monika's assistants and her husband in interpreting Monika's wishes and preferences, this conclusion was based on Monika's body language, that is, on how happy and relaxed she appeared, how alert and awake she was, and if she smiled – or clenched her teeth hard.

In contrast, Tage's wife seemed more oriented towards Tage as the person he is today with his current cognitive and physical shortcomings than towards restoring his 'old' identity or them as a couple. However, she was very resolute on what she valued when choosing personal assistants for Tage. When asked about what she considered as the personal assistants' primary task, she answered without hesitation:

Wife: To like Tage. It is ... and then the rest just follows. The most important thing is that they like him. It is most important. And then the rest follows. And they should kind of ... well show their love. They ... well like many of the girls do, they hug him and kiss him. It is important. And then you notice that he feels good. What is most important is that he is content. And then the purely practical tasks, it's obviously ... it will follow by itself. But if you do not like Tage, then this is not the right place for you.

She also stressed the importance of Tage having the opportunity to try new things and develop skills that he had not had the opportunity to develop earlier in life – like painting. Tage's assistants also talked about drawing and painting, which Tage currently engaged in regularly and which had been introduced by another assistant who was very interested in drawing and painting himself.

While not as immediately obvious as in the case of Monika and her husband, the efforts Tage's wife invested in finding the 'right' assistants could also be considered as a form of biographical work in the sense of consisting of actions aimed at achieving a sense of control and balance in her own, as well as Tage's, life. Additionally, her way of promoting the introduction of new activities in Tage's life, as well as the assistants' introducing such activities, could be understood as a way of giving the wife's as well as Tage's life meaning despite the illness and the changes it brings (compare with Corbin and Strauss 1988). Presumably, introducing new activities to Tage that he seemed to enjoy and was good at, despite his current extensive bodily and cognitive shortcomings, also added meaning to the work as a personal assistant.

The overarching everyday work that implied that extensive time and efforts were directed towards interpreting bodily and facial language and sounds may also be considered as a form of biographical work in the sense of being a way of supporting a person who no longer is able to tell about her wishes and preferences to remain self-determinant and able to influence his or her life to the extent possible in the current situation. This kind of everyday and biographical work is clearly in line with the ideology of disability activism and policy regarding the role of personal assistants. Research on personal assistance (e.g. Ungerson, 1999) has shown that personal aides of people with physical disabilities adopt this ideology of self-determination as a norm and consider it to be their duty to (only) act as the so-called assistance users' arms and legs. However, in the case of Monika and Tage, the personal assistants acted as (persistent and confident) interpreters of Tage's and Monika's will, preferences and desires, rather than as their arms and legs.

Lastly, one must acknowledge the efforts that both Monika's and Tage's spouses had invested, and still invested, in restoring biographical continuity in their own and their spouses' lives by keeping their spouses at home. In a way, Monika, Tage and their spouses could be considered as privileged by being entitled to personal assistance, as most people with dementia with similar care needs in Sweden do not have this opportunity but live in residential care. However, getting and having personal assistance also implied work for the spouses, such as applying for personal assistance from the very beginning, monitoring the assistance, hiring new assistants, etc. For both the persons with dementia and their spouses, it also meant that they had to accept that their home turned into a workplace for personal assistants. And, as told by Tage's wife, it was not necessarily the case that a person who she considered as qualified to be a good assistant for Tage was a great match for her:

Wife: Well it is not always that the assistant and myself match. But that's not the important thing. The important thing is, after all, that Tage gets the care he should have and that the assistant and Tage matches. That is how it is.

Interviewer: Mm. So you like ... you set your own needs aside ...?

Wife: Yes, I have to of course. For it is ... the assistant is hired to care for Tage.

What can we learn?

This chapter has aimed at showing the importance of relationships with and support from other people in order for people with dementia to sustain a sense of agency and self throughout the process. Dementia is a syndrome and includes a number of different diagnoses. Each specific dementia diagnosis, for example Alzheimer's disease, seemingly has a uniform trajectory and might be described in terms of stages. However, the diagnosis needs to be looked upon as 'both unity and diversity' (Gubrium & Lynott, 1985). Dementia could also be treated as a *chronic illness,* an illness to which the person living with the dementia and his or her family must accommodate and adjust. Using a chronic illness perspective on dementia allows us to work more explicitly with different features shared with other chronic illnesses. Not least, applying Corbin and Strauss's particular conceptualisation framework highlights that people with dementia as well as their carers actually have to *do* a lot of work in order to manage the illness trajectory. It also supports an understanding of the relationship between the ill and the well. Furthermore, abstracting the work done by ill individuals facilitates comparisons – for seeing similarities as well as differences – between groups of people with chronic illnesses (Conrad, 1987). In other words, these comparisons highlight 'both unity and diversity in the disease and its experience' (Gubrium & Lynott, 1985, p. 350).

Lastly, the chapter points to the importance of a tailored and individualised support for people with dementia in order to prevent *excess disabilities* exemplified by personal assistance.

References

Ballenger, J. F. (2006). Progress in the history of Alzheimer's disease: Importance of the context. *Journal of Alzheimer's Disease, 9,* 5–13.

Bartlett, R. & O'Connor, D. (2007). From personhood to citizenship: Broadening the lens for dementia practice and research. *Journal of Aging Studies, 21,* 107–118.

Behuniak, S. M. (2011). The living dead? The construction of people with Alzheimer's disease as zombies. *Ageing & Society, 31,* 70–92.

Boeije, H. R., Duijnstee, M. S. H., Grypdonck, M. H. F. & Pool, A. (2002). Encountering the downward phase: Biographical work in people with multiple sclerosis living at home. *Social Science & Medicine, 55,* 881–893.

Boyle, G. (2008). The Mental Capacity Act 2005: Promoting the citizenship of people with dementia? *Health and Social Care in the Community, 16,* 529–537.

Brody, E. M., Kleban, M. H., Lawton, M. P. & Silverman, H. A. (1971). Excess disabilities of mentally impaired aged: Impact of individualized treatment. *The Gerontologist, 11,* 124–133.

Conrad, P. (1987). The experience of illness: Recent and new directions. In J. Roth & P. Conrad (Eds.), *Research in the Sociology of Health Care,* Vol. 6. Greenwich, CT: JAI Press.

Corbin, J. M. & Strauss, A. (1985). Managing chronic illness at home: Three lines of work. *Qualitative Sociology, 8,* 224–247.

Corbin, J. M. & Strauss, A. (1988). *Unending Work and Care: Managing Chronic Illness at Home.* San Francisco: Jossey Bass.

Fox, P. (1989). From senility to Alzheimer's disease: The rise of the Alzheimer's disease movement. *The Milbank Quarterly, 67,* 58–102.

Gubrium, J. F. (1987). Structuring and destructuring the course of illness: The Alzheimer's disease experience. *Sociology of Health and Illness, 9,* 1–24.

Gubrium, J. F. & Lynott, R. J. (1985). Alzheimer's disease as biographical work. In W. A. Peterson & J. Quadagno (Eds.), *Social Bonds in Later Life: Aging and Interdependence.* Beverly Hills: Sage Publications.

Harnett, T. (2010). Seeking exemptions from nursing home routines: Residents' everyday influence attempts and institutional order. *Journal of Aging Studies, 24,* 292–301.

Hellström, I., Nolan, M. & Lundh, U. (2005). Awareness context theory and the dynamics of dementia: Improving understanding using emergent fit. *Dementia: The International Journal of Social Research and Practice, 4,* 269–295.

Hellström, I. (2009). Dignity and elderly spouses with dementia. In L. Nordenfelt (Eds.), *Dignity in Care for Older People.* Oxford: Blackwell – Wiley.

Jacques, A. (1988). *Understanding Dementia.* Edinburgh: Churchill Livingstone.

Jönson, H. & Taghizadeh Larsson, A. (2009). The exclusion of older people in disability activism and policies – a case of inadvertent ageism? *Journal of Aging Studies, 23,* 69–77.

Kahn, R. S. (1965). Comments. In M. P. Lawton & F. G. Lawton (Eds.), *Mental Impairment in the Aged* (pp. 109–114). Philadelphia: Philadelphia Geriatric Center.

Keady, J. (1999). *The dynamics of dementia: A modified grounded theory study.* Unpublished PhD dissertation. Bangor: University of Wales.

Kelly, F. & Innes, A. (2013). Human rights, citizenship and dementia care nursing. *International Journal of Older People Nursing, 8,* 61–70.

Kitwood, T. (1988). The technical, the personal, and the framing of dementia. *Social Behaviour, 3*, 161–179.

Kitwood, T. (1997). *Dementia reconsidered: The person comes first.* Buckingham: Open University Press.

Lobo, A., Launer, L., Fratiglioni, L., Andersen, K., Carlo, A. D., Breteler, M. et al. (2000). Prevalence of dementia and major subtypes in Europe: A collaborative study of population-based cohorts. Neurologic Diseases in the Elderly Research Group. *Neurology, 54*(11 Suppl 5), 4–9.

Nedlund, A.-C. & Nordh, J. (2015). Crafting citizen(ship) for people with dementia: How policy narratives at national level in Sweden informed politics of time from 1975 to 2013. *Journal of Aging Studies, 34*, 123–133.

Newton, R. D. (1948). The identity of Alzheimer's disease and senile dementia and their relationship to senility. *The British Journal of Psychiatry, 94*, 225–249.

Örulv, L. (2012). Reframing dementia in Swedish self-help group conversations: Constructing citizenship. *The International Journal of Self-help and Self-care, 6*, 9–41.

Österholm, J. H. & Hydén, L. C. (2014). Citizenship as practice: Handling communication problems in encounters between persons with dementia and social workers. *Dementia, 15*, 1457–1473. doi:10.1177/1471301214563959

Rogers, J. C., Holm, M. B., Burgio, L. D., Hsu, C, Hardin, J. M. & McDowell, B. J. (2000). Excess disability during morning care in nursing home residents with dementia. *International Psychogeriatrics, 12*, 267–282.

Sabat, S. R. (1994). Excess disability and malignant social psychology: A case study of Alzheimer's disease. *Journal of Community & Applied Social Psychology, 4*, 157–166.

Strauss, A. L., Corbin, J., Fagerhaugh, S., Glaser, B. G., Maines, D., Suczek, C. & Wiener, C. L. (1984). *Chronic Illness and the Quality of Life.* St. Louis: Mosby.

Ungerson, C. (1999). Personal assistants and disabled people: An examination of a hybrid form of work and care. *Work, Employment & Society, 13*, 583–600.

van den Akker, M., Buntinx, F., Metsemakers, J. F. M., Roos, S. & Knottnerus, J. A. (1998). Multimorbidity in general practice: Prevalence, incidence, and determinants of co-occurring chronic and recurrent diseases. *Journal of Clinical Epidemiology, 51*, 367–75.

Ville, I. (2005). Biographical work and returning to employment following a spinal cord injury. *Sociology of Health & Illness, 27*, 324–350.

Williams, S. (2000). Chronic illness as biographical disruption or biographical disruption as chronic illness? Reflections on a core concept. *Sociology of Health & Illness, 22*, 40–67.

9

'HOME IS SOMEWHERE IN-BETWEEN-PASSAGE': THE STORIES OF RELOCATION TO A RESIDENTIAL HOME BY PERSONS WITH DEMENTIA

Parvin Pooremamali

One of the most critical life transitions for older people is moving into residential care that requires major changes from living an active and independent life (Aminzadeh et al., 2009; Lee et al., 2013). In fact, persons with dementia experienced the transition as a passage to a new life stage that often resulted in occupational deprivation. Transitions include a particular spatial expression of aging and care because of a shift from active to passive, from good to poor health, from caregiver to care recipient (Milligan, 2012). Various disciplinary viewpoints, including sociological, anthropological and psychological, attempt to understand the concept of home for people in late life (Cutchin, 2013; Oswald & Wahl, 2005). Home is, in other words, the place of most significant attachment and meanings that has an important role in older adults' ongoing lives (Rowles, 2003). Hence, it should not be viewed as a constrained venue but as a space of ongoing daily contact with the community (Haak, 2006; Rowles, 2008). Home therefore is a complex blend of emotional, cognitive, behavioural and social bonds, and the factors that generate a feeling of home include privacy, control, autonomy, connection and family (Cooney, 2012). However, the concept of home has different meanings in every culture at different stages of life and is affected by different conditions and circumstances (Oswald & Wahl, 2005).

Indeed, several researchers have recently highlighted the meaning of home as a crucial element in the process of relocation to another place, for example from home to home or from home into an assisted-living or residential care facility (Oswald & Wahl, 2005). According to Seamon (1980), people are attached to place and create meaning both bodily and emotionally through association with the regularity and routine of everyday activity. There are a number of studies on habitation and the elderly, recognizing how continuity with old life and routine, preserving personal identity, security, comfort, control and belonging are significant elements in shaping a meaning of home (Cooney, 2012; Cutchin, 2013). As a result, understanding the meaning of home among persons with dementia requires seeing how the notion of meaning of home is understood by different disciplines. For example, from an environmental psychology perspective, Hayward (1975) suggested home has a meaning in relation to physical structure as a space, as a locus in space and self-identity and as a social and cultural unit. From this framework, the meaning of home involves a transactional relationship between persons, activities and environment that changes over time (Oswald & Wahl, 2005). In addition, several studies have underlined the relational aspects of the meaning of home, arguing that the meaning of home is a dynamic relationship between the person and the environment. In such composition, the meaning of home is often enacted through meaningful activities (Wenger, 1998).

Other work has reinforced the importance of the transaction between the person and the environment and has highlighted that meaning is constantly negotiated, or reconstructed, through the continual re-coordination of person and place (Shank & Cutchin, 2010). From this perspective, the meaning of home is generated from daily life activities that occur in familiar places within a temporal framework encapsulated in the concept of habituation (Altman et al., 1992). Thus, home modifications and adaptation may positively affect the meaning of home as a place of security, safety and comfort. In addition, decreasing the demands of the environment and supporting the continuation of habitual routines or rituals could link older people to their homes and thereby reinforce identity, self-esteem and control (Tanner et al., 2008).

The psychological and social psychological approaches attempt to explain the meaning of home in terms of deep-rooted psychological needs for identity, control, privacy, security, intimacy and social status. Moreover, environmental gerontology has focused attention on concepts such as aging in place and place attachment, particularly in assessing the suitability and familiarity of places and how older people conceptualize later life and give meaning to the home. In taking this approach, the meaning of home is viewed as a set of experiences and feelings about a geographic location that emotionally bind a person to home and involves the interactive relationship or bonding between a person and the setting that occurs over time and helps people make sense of the world and move on (Chaudhury, 2008; Oswald & Wahl, 2005). Thus, the meaning of home constantly changes because it is linked to experiences under different situations and contexts (Lewin, 2001).

Finally, the phenomenological and developmental approach highlights the meaning of home as stability and continuity and seeks to understand the changes in the meaning of home during the course of a person's lifetime (Somerville, 1997).

Although one of the most critical life transitions for older people is moving into residential care, remarkably little is known about how to make meaningful the identity transition for persons with dementia belonging to ethnic minority groups who are moved into non-cultural- and non-linguistic-based residential homes. Furthermore, little is known about what makes living in a residential care facility meaningful or meaningless and whether participation in daily life activities provides the persons with dementia a sense of continuity in life and reconstruction of identity.

Hence, the aim of this chapter is to understand the perceptions of 'becoming and being at home' in residential care facilities among persons with dementia who belong to ethnic minorities, how they attempt to be integrated in their new home and what influences these perceptions.

In this chapter I focus on two persons with dementia, a woman and a man, belonging to different ethnic minority groups in Sweden, who lived within two bounded areas (residential care homes) and were subject to rules and restrictions not of their own choosing. The woman lived in a residential home for persons with dementia with all the medical and technical resources of a nursing home rather than large assisted-living facilities, and the man lived in a special dementia homelike-care unit that was integrated within a nursing home facility.

I used a case-study design, with narrative interviews and narrative analysis. These participants were selected through family members based on the following inclusion criteria: (1) having a diagnosis of dementia according to the *Diagnostic and Statistical Manual of Mental Disorders (DSM-5®)* (American Psychiatric Association, 2013); (2) age 65 years old or older to capture the geriatric perspective; and (3) ability to communicate. I then met the individuals to ascertain their interest in participating in this study and set up an initial meeting with them and their designated family members. The initial meeting provided the opportunity to establish rapport, answer questions about the study process and obtain informed consent and assent. Individuals with cognitive impairment may not have the capacity for consent but can give assent or verbal agreement to participate in a study. Family members' active involvement in the study was limited to the consent process, although at one interview, a family caregiver was present at the participant's request. This was acceptable to provide the participant with psychological comfort and security. Prior to each interview, the researcher spent 10–15 minutes in general conversation with the participant to build rapport and ease any apprehension. The interviews began with conversation about their experiences, feelings and thoughts about their transition and relocation from home to the residential care facility and their daily life activities, needs, desires, obstacles and expectations as well. Moreover, I asked them to talk about the ways they manage their habitual activities and the ways they cope with circumstances in the new home.

Case description

Hamed (pseudonym) is an 81-year-old immigrant man from Iraq who has lived more than 20 years in Sweden. He was admitted to a residential home for persons with dementia from a psychiatric hospital, where he had been treated for symptoms associated with dementia and aggression. The residential home was located in an unfamiliar neighborhood far from Hamed's former accommodation. In this home, relationships were seen as functional, staff members were focused on completing tasks and it was not a space for personal and supportive relationships. As a retired immigrant, Hamed was an active and healthy man and very fit. He enjoyed helping his wife with daily life activities (shopping and preparing food, cleaning, walking, and watching TV, etc.). He had a very attractive personality with a sense of humor that was catching. He strongly identified with his Muslim heritage. He previously always lived in a segregated neighborhood, predominantly with Muslim neighbours. Hamed used to go to mosque daily in the morning to participate in prayer with his friends. There he remained until the shops opened. On the way home, he would go to the local grocery stores to buy ingredients for the dish of the day that his wife recommended and requested. He always walked to the mosque and back home. He often had other people as company on the way home. He was very determined to make decisions about everything and have control over his and his wife's life wherever he was and whoever might try to diminish his power and control. This was the most significant problem in providing a safe environment for him to live.

When Hamed moved to the residential home, he was fixated that he had to go to the mosque and perform his daily ritual early in the morning. He was so determined that every morning, he changed his outfit, picked up his hat and stick and was ready to go to the mosque. He tried to go through the corridor and open the door as he did in his home. When the staff stopped him, he became very agitated and aggressive, and often staff members took hard and undesirable action to take him forcibly back to his room. Once he went out and walked for miles and was not able to find his way back. This created a significant care management problem, as the residential home had no bilingual staff to communicate with him. He would also wander at night and become very disoriented and enter other residents' rooms. This was very distressing for the other residents. However, a variety of care management options, such as increasing the neuroleptic medication and locking his room, were applied and had side effects, which affected his movement and coordination. In addition, he became very agitated and aggressive when he could not open his door. He was restless and bitter and upset about his situation in the residential home. He insisted that he wanted to go back home.

Sonia is an 85-year-old woman who immigrated from Chile and has lived for more than 30 years in Sweden. She is able to reflect upon and articulate her experiences before, during, and after her move to the residential home. She moved to the residential home because she was not taking care of herself and because of general loneliness (her husband had died two years before). She had four children, who lived in the same city. She did not seem an unhappy person by nature. She described staff at her residence as very kind, helpful and respectful and was happy that some staff members were immigrants, especially one who speaks Spanish. She strongly identified with her atheism and always lived in integrated neighborhoods and did not live in predominantly immigrant quarters. She is in a residential care facility for persons with dementia, where relationships with staff members were both functional and personal. Supportive relationships also existed within the home, and the personnel fostered more expressive and personal relationships. She was able to anticipate and prepare for the move to the residential home. Consequently, she entered the residential home with a positive attitude for living at ease.

My new home is somewhere-in-between passage

My new home is somewhere-in-between passage. (Sonia)

As a core theme, 'New home somewhere-in-between passage' was a metaphoric quotation about a passage between past, present and future. During this passage, Sonia and Hamed moved through a life trajectory that encompassed a turning point of many changes in daily life conditions that sequentially required new patterns of actions and coping strategies to recapture meanings in life. Nevertheless, four superordinate themes exist in relation to home: 'Home is a place of the daily life habitual activities'; 'Home evokes a recollection of experiences of relating being-with-others'; 'Home is a place of constructing and reconstruction of the new selves' and 'The new home is the end of an active and independent life'.

Home is a place of the daily life habitual activities was about Hamed's and Sonia's challenges of preserving continuity in daily habitual activities and rituals and how doing the ordinary things and personal rhythms have changed in their *new home*. It seemed that recapturing and reconstructing the meaning of home in the residential home created challenges that become more difficult as the environmental competence of these persons declined. For example, Hamed's relation between feelings of home was affected by his engagement in daily spiritual practice and the places (mosque and home) through which he constructed and reconstructed meanings. Hamed described the importance of daily prayer, a practice that Hamed had continued in mosques and at home since coming to Sweden. Hamed showed his holy Quran and kissed the Quran with specific ritualistic respect and then stated:

I have prayed whole my life in the mosque and every night in my home and I always felt better after I did that. It gave me hope, and I prayed to be better with my illness. ... I could no longer read the holy Quran, but other persons used to read and recite it to me and I heard and listened to them and it gave me happiness. ... I cannot read it longer and it make me sad. Reading the holy Quran always gave me hope to cope with my weakness, sorrow, pain. I prayed God to not be dependence to my children and not to be placed to a home with strangers.... Who did not share the same faith as we Muslim did.... Here I am disrupted to contact with my God, especially in the morning.... Different persons are coming in my room and going out from my room.... They are men and women and they disrupt and bother me.... But I continue to pray in order to receive more power to deal with all disruptions moments and accept my life here....

It seemed that both Hamed's abilities and the environment led to a lack of routine in relation to his habitual activity, causing difficulty in his ability to manage the new situation. In addition, the transition to his new home encompassed endings and disruptions in maintaining continuity in identity, relationships and environment that led to a lack of ability to be integrated into the new home as a whole. As a result, Hamed experienced the new home as losses of autonomy, self-determination, choices and the opportunity to grow spiritually. Hamed pointed out how belonging to a mosque linked him to his past and provided an avenue for him to keep himself in touch with his past life and see himself as a member in the mosque community. He said,

I've been involved in the mosque most of my life, especially in Sweden. I grow up with my spiritual ritual and it means too much to my identity as a Muslim. I enjoyed being with others landsmen and do not feel myself alone. ... Everything was different in the mosque ... and I miss it, my landsmen, the praying together, shaking hands, hugging together, closeness, supporting, strengthen the soul and the soul tranquillity and all the social things ....

McColgan (2005) described how identity is linked to home (place) and, especially, the importance of home as a place of privacy and choice. When living in a nursing home, the extent of group control, shadowing and routines can stand in the way of this reconstruction of the past, gaining privacy and maintaining autonomy and choice. Residents have to resist actively these elements of nursing home culture in order to construct a reality based upon personal values. In fact, habit establishment and reconstruction are essential dimensions of developing a sense of belonging and a rhythm of interactions in and out of place, which in turn lead to becoming at home in a residential home (Cutchin, 2013). According to Dewey, all human action is based on habits (Dewey 1992/1957 in Cutchin, 2013). The life stories of Hamed and Sonia illustrate how habits function as automatic responses to environmental stimuli. According to Kielhofner (2008), habits are patterns of behavior that are often performed spontaneously and often need only low-level conscious effort and thought to engage in and accomplish. Thus, performing habitual activity releases thoughts for other things. In addition, habits depend on a familiarity with the environment that allows people to internalise rules for behavior. The case of Hamed sheds light on the claim by Kielhofner (2008) concerning the importance of environment: it can provide opportunities and resources for activities whilst also placing demands and constraints that hinder people's ability to respond in habitual ways. In fact, despite living with dementia, Hamed sought to retain continuity in his spiritual life and tried to stay in contact with his spiritual community.

Research studies indicate that spiritual activity can improve health and emotional well-being. Thus, spirituality is an important activity for adapting to and coping with memory loss, preserving self-worth and maintaining a sense of normalcy for older persons with dementia (Beuscher & Grando, 2009; Carr, Hicks-Moore & Montgomery, 2011; Clare, 2002; Narayanasamy, 2002). The case of Hamed may confirm the aforementioned studies claiming that spiritual practices not only connect individuals with personal faith, but also provide vital connections with other people and possibly a sense of belonging and identity for persons with dementia. As a result, Hamed's spiritual activity habit was socially constructed and developed through connection to the integrated systems of activity that guide thoughts, values and behaviours (Dewey, 1957, p. 39 in Cutchin, 2013).

On the contrary, Sonia experienced opportunities for her growth in a way that she could engage in exploring, redefining and preserving new meanings. Previous meanings in relation to her daily habitual activities that were not applicable when she lived in her own home could flourish. Her expectation of habitual activities was modified and negotiated or replaced with one that was realistic for the new situation and in a way that Sonia could regain a sense of control and mastery.

Perhaps the most obvious reason for Sonia's integration into her new home was that the opportunities in her new home made it possible to maintain continuities, specifically her habitual body- and beauty-management activities. These continuities facilitated reconstruction of meaning and coping with changes that fostered her ability to enjoy her life and integrate into her new home. Sonia pointed at her vanity and make-up table in the corner of her living room and in faltering words explained:

> I just sit there and look me in the mirror. It makes me feel good. It's something that I like, I love it and it brought me pleasure. So I just want to keep being able to fix my hair and do things, and, that's all, really.

Sonia described in particular how the physical appearance of other older adults in the residential home provoked her interest in body image and appearance-management activities intended to improve, maintain or alter one's body or body image. She said:

> It was a long time ago as I fixed my hair ... I saw fine ladies here in the dining room ... and they reminded me when I fixed my hair. ... It did not feel good to be unkempt.

I also want to be dressed fine here and then I talked to my daughter and she then they fixed everything here ... beauty was always important to me ... I always followed the fashion and himself used to sew my beautiful clothes. ... I always cared for my body and beauty .... and then I asked my son to take me to the mall where I bought an expensive perfume that I always used it in my life. ... I want to smell well.

This citation shed light on the claim by Dewey (in Cutchin, 2013) that habits are shaped through our ongoing involvement in place, such as social interaction and activities of daily living. In fact, these cases shed light on Dewey's argument about habits as central functions of Hamed's and Sonia's continuous transactions with their world. In other words, Hamed's and Sonia's degree of integration and adaptation to the residential home depended on how they could coordinate with their new home through the development and use of their previous habitual activities. This confirmed the claim by Dewey about how the nature, structure and quality of a place provide the opportunity to develop or improve habits and enable a person's thought, movement and other forms of action to respond to a situation and its emerging challenges. In fact, the transition to a new home included both losses and opportunities for Sonia and Hamed, but it depended on a fit between person and environment that either facilitated or limited the continuity trajectories in relation to daily habitual activities. This is in line with Cutchin's (2013) argument that the meaning of becoming at-home is 'a holistic, continuous matter that varies by person, is both enjoyed and suffered, and include the continuity of life before, during, and after the move' (p. 105).

Home evokes a recollection of experiences of relating: Being-with-others was the second theme describing different challenges Hamed and Sonia encountered in making the transition from home to a residential care facility. Feelings of abandonment and loss of home, ritual, lifestyle and the opportunities for contact with friends and relatives were a large part of their narratives. In essence, then, Sonia was able to construct the residential home as home, while Hamed had significant difficulty in viewing the residential home positively as home. As a result, meanings of home and meanings of the residential home were infinitely different for these individuals. As these cases showed, Sonia's and Hamed's experiences with other people, in past and current places, seemed to play an important role in creating a sense of belonging to their residential home. It seems that the physical layout and location of the particular residential home and the familiarity of the neighborhood played a significant role in each individual's sense of belonging to the new home. For example, for Sonia, the new home became a place where the familiar outside environment, the view through the window outside towards the street and shopping mall and proximity to her previous home and her children afforded typical memories, happiness, security and a sense of belonging. It perhaps served better as an adaptive ability for Sonia to maintain tranquility, control and comfort in being in the new home. Consequently, the findings highlight an important question regarding the transaction between environment and person in the meaning of home and how the individual's meaning of home may reflect behavioral adaptations in the new home. On the contrary, Hamed had no past memories and feelings about the new home before moving in. Hamed viewed his transition into the residential care facility as cause for disrupting his habits in performing religious rituals. Specifically, he pointed to dissatisfaction with the residential home because of the limitation and disruption of his freedom to perform the habitual ways of this activity. Perhaps being a part of daily prayer in the mosque was a means through which Hamed could express who he is to himself and to others.

However, a crucial piece in the basis of engagement between self and place is the set of habitual actions that ties together not only place and self but also consciousness and the body, mind and other and even memory and imagination, in line with Dewey. In other words, habitus is basically linked to the rootedness and a sense of home because the activities that people make on the basis of their habitus are consciously experienced and chosen (Casey, 2001). As a result, people are able to foster a conscious sense of home. However, the case of Hamed revealed how internal and external obstacles to performing habitual activities may diminish integration into a residential home. As a result, meaning is an essential component of human experiences, derived in daily life through many habitual activities. Thus, maintaining habitual activities and maintaining meanings are both vulnerable to the process of transition from home to a residential home (Shank & Cutchin, 2010). Moreover, both persons associated a feeling of 'belonging' with feeling at home. 'Belonging' was defined as becoming at home and being part of the group and experienced as a sense of commonality, companionship, relaxation and fun. Hamed's and Sonia's stories about their homes, their locations and the objects physically, metaphorically and narratively within invoke different meanings. For example, Sonia addressed the symbolic meaning associated with the location of the residential home and its subsequent meanings. She talked about her memory of the neighborhood from when she used to walk with her husband to the shopping mall, and it reminded her of her husband when he was alive. On the contrary, Hamed had no memories associated with the home or with the neighbourhood. He talked about being a stranger in a strange city and country. However, this part of the narrative shed light on the following: 'Dewey's central tenets of continuity, contingency, situation, and action present a worldview that focuses on holistic relations being constantly remade by activity (transactions) to address ongoing change' (Cutchin et al., 2003, p. 235).

Moreover, considering the relation between meaning of home and objects, the findings confirmed the importance of being surrounded by objects filled with past memories that make it possible for older people to combine the past and the present in their day-to-day lives, in line with Jackson (1996). Having a familiar neighbourhood might well be explained as a mediated factor to Sonia's ability to cope with an increasingly chaotic world as the dementia progresses (Greenwood et al., 2001). This confirmed the claim by Jackson (1996) describing the role of objects in construction of meaning and a sense of continuity. Likewise, transitional objects (Loboprabhu, Molinari & Lomax, 2007) seem to act as 'anchors and mediators' to Sonia in the period of uncertainty. Cutchin (2007) argued that the combined external and internal dimensions of home create a material and symbolic landscape that mediates the social and individual habit process. In fact, each of these residential homes contained specific physical, social, cultural and historical dimensions as a component of self, in line with Rowles (1991). For example, Sonia developed memories of her environment that imbued locations of specific happenings with emotional meaning, allowing her to better immerse herself within the places of the past to transcend the limitation of the present, linking who she has been to who she is as described by others (Kuo, 2011).

According to Cutchin (2013), our relationship with place has both depths of meaning and complexity; home and the experience of it is a process that is both personal and social, tangled with selfhood and with the larger social and historical contexts. Moreover, the findings shed light on Shank and Cutchin's (2010) discourse about how meaning depends on many factors and reflects the complexity of relationship between person and place, past and present, objects and experiences, all of which change with time. Habits are always shaped through our ongoing involvement in place (Cutchin, 2013), and so the findings may provide knowledge about the role of place in these two persons' lives that may be useful for other older people's relationship and integration with place. In this regard, Sonia's and Hamed's life stories may increase our knowledge of which housing forms and home environments are most appropriate to offer elderly immigrants, considering their cultural and social background, that is, which form of habitation they prefer (Lewin, 2001). Therefore, in accordance with Rowles and Ravdal (2002) and Cutchin et al. (2003), additional study is needed to describe and explain the relationships of person, place and action of people with dementia under transition from home to a residential care facility.

The findings also demonstrate how Sonia and Hamed reaffirmed a sense of self through negotiating role capacity and role identity in the face of a changing habitual activity in the new home. However, the findings confirmed Christiansen's (1999) argument concerning how the loss or change of occupation related to identity is particularly challenging during aging. As the findings indicate, Sonia's and Hamed's everyday lives in relation to their past habitual activities need to be understood from a life-course perspective. As their life stories demonstrate, habitual activities offer, in particular, channels for obtaining role maintenance in relation to other people. This sheds light on the claim by Lemon et al. (1972) about how confirming responses of others is important for confirming role identities. Thus, a change of habitual activities may lead to a subsequent risk that role identities will not be affirmed and also lead to losses of identity.

In sum, the concept of 'doing' for Hamed encompassed daily prayer in the mosque while he struggled to maintain a sense of 'being' that is personally meaningful to him. Praying in the mosque is associated with a sense of being because Hamed described this kind of 'being' in terms of having time and tranquility to reflect, rediscover the self, enjoy the moment and enjoy being with people and freely and actively choose activities according to his revised values and priorities of life (Hammell, 2004). In addition, Hamed's emphasis on going to the mosque seemed to be a need for a sense of 'belonging' that reveals the importance of relationships and connectedness for a continuity of his social identity. Belonging within a context (residential home) can underpin both the ability to do and contribute to the pleasure and meaningfulness of doing (Hammell, 2004). And a search for 'becoming' through spiritual activity in the mosque perhaps generated an opportunity for Hamed to reassess his life priorities to explore new opportunities about who or what he wishes to become through reflecting on values, selecting priorities, making choices and engaging in activities over the course of the dementia trajectory, in line with Hammell (2004).

Home is a place of constructing and reconstruction of the new selves is the third theme regarding the relationship between the feeling of home and the attributes and processes of the self. In fact, Sonia and Hamed were differently engaged in exploring the meaning of the transition and in finding new meanings in their new homes. It seems that the process of creating and redefining identity and self was complex dependent on the degree of factors that either recognized or resisted Sonia's and Hamed's expectations and restructuring of life routines and habits in a way that was somehow congruent with the new situation and allowed the person to continue his or her habitual activities.

The home is seen as an extension of oneself, perhaps in two senses, as a distinction can be made between the subjective self (the 'I') and the objective self ('Me'). The first region concerns the ongoing processes that basically constitute the self, those desires, feelings, hopes and actions in the context, in accordance with Chaudhury (2008). For example, Hamed said the following:

> I do not feel this place is mine and I am not belonging to this home. My home had no snow. … It is warm and light … I am a stranger here because.

In fact, the meaning of home for Hamed may embrace home as a physical structure, as a place, as a locus in space, as self and self-identity and as a social, cultural and religious unit in line with place-attachment theory (Schumaker & Taylor, 1983). As this case showed, a lack of the sense of being, becoming and belonging-at-home appeared when Hamed talked about his feeling of not being a part of the new home. On the contrary, Sonia felt relaxed and comfortable in her new home because of new stimuli and meaning and the availability of services that helped her with managing her personal care. She said:

> I saw this that all residents have nice clothes on and is fine in the hair. ... It seems they are going to a party. ... It reminds me my own life and the way as I was before ... I always cared very much to my beauty with fixing my hair, nails, face and wearing me nice clothes. ... I used to sew nice clothes for me ... but then I get sick, I could not longer to fix those things as I was used to doing. ... It is very pleasant for me to feel nice and fresh again....

In fact, Sonia was able to construct and reconstruct the experience of a self grounded in the continuity of her life course in relation to body- and beauty-management activities. Maintaining her body image seemed to be an essential aspect of Sonia's identity and self that in turn mediated her integration in becoming and being at home. Nevertheless, when considering developing identity in residential care, it is assumed that each person may have a different perception of meaning in developing a new identity in a new place and context. However, shifts in meaning of home are influenced by factors such as resources in the family, the cultural, physical, and social environment, accessibility, attitudes and social organization, which in turn provide opportunities to redefine the self through a feeling of competence and mastery as well as through perception of others in context. Moreover, constructing and reconstructing a new identity depends on adjusting to a life situation, for instance in a residential home and as a person with dementia facing challenges, and adaptive strategies shifted. For example, through choices, personal autonomy and support of others (caregivers), they may compensate for the activities they have lost with others that generate meaning and thus have the possibility to master an ongoing changing life. In addition, the cases revealed how regaining identity was connected to how daily life practices are seen in the person's cultural values, norms and roles, as well as the degree of possibilities in the residential care facility that support and enable the person to tie together their past, present and future life. Overall findings in line with Hasselkus (2002) and Hammell (2004) demonstrated habitual activity is more than doing.

Thus, understanding the meaning attached to home on negotiating identities requires a holistic consideration of the complex transaction between the environmental context and the person during life-course trajectories (Larson & Zemeke, 2003).

The new home is the end of an active and independent life is the fourth theme. Sonia and Hamed expressed different views about the meaning of their relocation to the residential care facility. For example, for Sonia, relocation symbolized the end of an active and independent life and the passage to a more protected and supported life. She described how her life with other old and fragile persons led to awareness of her own vulnerable health conditions and the reality that she is not able to continue her daily life activities as she did before.

I need care as these aged and sick people. ... I could not make food and feed myself. ... I could not go out. ... I could not fix my hair. ... I was afraid to be alone ... here I feel myself more secure....

On the contrary, for Hamed having freedom means doing what he wants to do in his own place and a supported space for supporting connection between himself and his family. Hamed defined home as a place to enable him to stay with his family as a unit and maintain emotional closeness between himself and his wife and children. Hence, he viewed moving to a residential care facility as an end to his life and to who he was and who he had been. He stated:

I have left a big part of my existence in my home....Here I do not exist even though I am alive. My life is not separated from my whole family my grandchildren and gran gram children

Hamed perceived the process of his relocation as a violation of his rights. He was disappointed and sorry that his children relocated him from his home to an unfamiliar home. He addressed their ignorance and responsibility in taking care of him according to the Islamic rule by referring to a quote from the Quran. According to Hamed, the relocation was forced on him and he had no opportunity to make decisions and exercise choice. In accordance with Aminzadeh et al. (2009; Aminzadeh, et al., 2010), Hamed and Sonia described their relocation from home to residential home as the end of an 'active and independent life', and the passage to some more protected, dependent and structured lifestyles when they faced disruption and alienation caused by dementia. For Sonia, home means the feeling of being secure, characterized by a caring atmosphere of warmth and comfort. She accepted the relinquishing of roles as something to be expected with age and accepted her new role as a care receiver. Thus, she did not feel loss when she could no longer carry out prior food-related activities. She said,

my frail condition made me more vulnerable and weak....My inner strength was failing and I fall and injured myself ... and I could no longer make and prepare my food and coffee even though I received help of my daughter and home services....

Moreover, for Sonia a feeling of home was connected with security, warmth and comfort, specifically those days when there was a Spanish-speaking staff member. Both Sonia and Hamed highlighted having a staff who could communicate in their own language. In addition, both mentioned the importance of living in a residential care facility in a familiar environment as a reason for the feeling of home. Sonia said,

I feel secure and receive help of personal who speak on my own language. I live very close to my previous home. ... I remember the street outside here and that mall as I used to go more often with my husband. ... Sometimes I miss him and wished if he was alive and we could walk to the mall....

Conclusion

The life stories of Sonia and Hamed revealed how home is an integral part of a person's identity and the perception of the meaning of a home involves a range of habitual practices. On the other hand, the findings shed light on a Deweyan place–person transaction perspective about the potential influences of reminiscence of place and habitual activities in regaining meaning of home (Cutchin, 2003). In addition, the findings highlighted the importance of the contextual and environmental conditions of the residences, such as the availability of emotional and instrumental supports according to a person's needs and expectations. Continuing habitual life activities and places are acknowledged as having mutual relationships to identity (Christiansen, 1999). In fact, the preservation of external continuity such as relationships, roles and activities over time contributes to a sense of consistency of personal identity (Atchley, 1989; Kaufman, 1988). For example, Hamed and Sonia described themselves in terms of their 'doing' abilities and disabilities and valued opportunities to continue their habitual life activities that reflected their personal identity. Moreover, these individuals reflected upon how their choices of habitual activities are associated with who they were before and who they are now. However, the stories of Sonia and Hamed showed how environment, place and limitations on and enrichment of habitual activities limit or promote a sense of becoming and being at a new home.

Nonetheless, in accordance with Cutchin (2013), the findings indicated the role of transferred habits and the role of imagination and habits of thoughts in facilitating or diminishing the sense of becoming and being at home. Thus, place integration can be facilitated by helping residents develop new habits of thought and activity. As a result, encouraging older people to utilize habits as tools to integrate with a new home must be accompanied by the development of residential home culture, environment and management that supports an integrative habitus.

As these cases demonstrated, the functional abilities of the person with dementia may be presented with a challenge to handle habitual life activities. For example, being ill because of dementia disability involves a transformation of people who consider themselves as capable to people who view themselves as fragile, weak and disabled. In a residential home, however, self and identity, along with participation in habitual activities, may play an essential role in construction and reconstruction of an adapted identity. In fact, if we want to understand the nation of identity among people with dementia living in a residential home, we must consider the relationship between the contextual patterns of a residential home and systems of meaning that may shape the behavior of a person with dementia and his or her engagement in the habitual activities and his or her sense of 'doing, being, becoming and belonging' in the new home. Indeed, through minimizing losses and focusing instead on abilities and the opportunity to gain personal meaning from everyday activities, consequences of dementia, as well as the experiences and the meaning of dementia, may be altered. Furthermore, both the cultural and relational milieu must be taken into account in order to understand how the person with dementia constructs and reconstructs her or his identity in the new home. Structures in residential care and systems of meaning, for instance, can either constrain or hamper a person-centred care by limiting or escalating the individuals' choices, as well as the impact or efficacy of their choices. These two systems always work together. Within this framework, we should understand the person's transition from home to residential home and how the person creates, recreates and alters her or his identity along the lines of possibility, accessibility, power and enabling features of the residential care at the same time as they may be constricted within the residential care facility's limits. In this way, we can explain the creation, recreation and transformation of identity through daily life practice within the social structure of the residential care home. For example, Sonia could better create and recreate her identity through the degree of choices and decision-making in being a part of her habitual life activities, which in turn increased opportunities for her in being and becoming an agent in what she is and does in everyday practice and to be integrated into the residential home. On the contrary, the case of Hamed revealed how being limited within the social structure of the residential care and lacking opportunity to perform habitual activities may lead to a lack of re-creation of identity and of integration into the residential home. In regard to such dilemmas we need to understand and explain what really happens to creation of a new identity in the absence or presence of opportunities in being part of the habitual life activities. In line with Christiansen (1999), the case of Sonia revealed how the experience of dementia was reduced when she was given an opportunity to gain personal meaning from habitual activities.

In fact, as these two case examples show, continuity in the desired habitual activity, choices and decision-making, personal autonomy and external resources and possibilities seemed to allow Hamed and Sonia to maintain an acceptable and satisfying sense of personal identity. For example, Sonia, through engagement in her past and desired habitual body- and beauty-management activities and discovery of new aspects of herself, interacted with others and reconstructed new habits, roles, routines and interests that in turn promoted a sense of continued growth and acceptable self-identity. In addition, Sonia may be integrated in the residential home through *being a part of her habitual activity* because of maintaining a sense of continuity of identity, a sense that she had earlier in life or prior to the onset of dementia and receiving a diagnosis. Thus, understanding how engagement in habitual activities generates meaning for a person and how transaction of place and person involves those activities and meanings is necessary. The culture and social structure of a residential home appear to have a strong influence on the range and quality of activities available as well as the security, level of personal attention and autonomy afforded to residents (Harmer & Orrell, 2008). For example, the care routines (activities of daily living or ADLs) that often occurred in the morning may take priority over a spiritual activity of a Muslim person, who is accustomed to pray and make his or her morning ritual. As a result, the residential context can have a significant effect on the behavior of a person when he or she is removed from familiar daily routines, home and family, which in turn creates a sense of isolation from society and affects the person's motivation to continue the daily life practices. These life stories shed light on Cooney's (2012) observations regarding the role of mediating factors, such as older people's adaptive responses, expectations and past experiences and the ethos of care, institutional culture and environment in the residential care facility, on a positive or negative feeling of home.

Implications and recommendations

In light of the findings, it is important to place persons with dementia who belong to ethnic minorities in culturally sensitive environments. For example, if we look for ways to adapt residential care housing for these persons in order to maintain daily independence, we should not ignore how spiritual activity affects well-being. As discussed earlier, persons with dementia belonging to ethnic minorities may experience greater vulnerabilities during the transition. Perhaps these persons need more emotional and instrumental support from the professional and family caregivers. The findings in agreement with Aminzadeh et al. (2009) indicate how a successful transition may depend not only on individual factors but also on the qualities and safety of the living environment. As a result, in order to establish a responsive system of care and affordable supportive-housing options, the heterogeneity of the older persons must be considered with regard to the diverse needs and preferences of the older populations.

The physical and social details that these two persons revealed about their current homes tell complicated stories and offer complex representations of their life-course experiences, personal, cultural and societal expectations and goals and the historical context that framed each person's life. In fact, meanings of home for these persons differ noticeably, illustrating the importance of applying a theoretical lens from an environmental-positioning perspective alongside a transactional perspective. In addition, the findings showed how the meaning of home is partly fluid and conditional (de Medeiros et al., 2013) and depends on the position of the social actors involved, which varies over time and circumstances.

References

American Psychiatric Association (2013). *Diagnostic and Statistical Manual of Mental Disorders (DSM-5®)*. Washington, DC Psychiatric Pub.

Aminzadeh, F., Dalziel, W. B., Molnar, F. J. & Garcia, L. J. (2009). Symbolic meaning of relocation to a residential care facility for persons with dementia. *Aging & Mental Health, 13*, 487–496.

Aminzadeh, F., Molnar, F. J., Dalziel, W. B. & Garcia, L. J. (2010). Meanings, functions, and experiences of living at home for individuals with dementia at the critical point of relocation. *Journal of Gerontological Nursing, 36*, 28–35.

Altman, I. & Low, S. (1992). *Human Behavior and Environments: Advances in Theory and Research*. V. 12, Place attachment. New York: Plenum Press.

Atchley, R. (1989). A continuity theory of normal aging. *Gerontologist, 29*, 183–190.

Beuscher, L. & Grando, V. T. (2009). Using spirituality to cope with early-stage Alzheimer's disease. *Western Journal of Nursing Research, 31*(5), 583–598.

Carr, T. J., Hicks-Moore, S. & Montgomery, P. (2011). What's so big about the 'little things': A phenomenological inquiry into the meaning of spiritual care in dementia. *Dementia, 10*, 399–414.

Casey, E. S. (2001). Body, self and landscape: A geophilosophical inquiry into the place-world. In P. C. Adams, S. Hoelscher & K. E. Till (Eds.), *Textures of Place: Exploring Humanist Geographies* (pp. 403–425). Minneapolis: University of Minnesota Press.

Chaudhury, H. (2008). *Remembering Home: Rediscovering the Self in Dementia*. Baltimore: Johns Hopkins University Press.

Christiansen, C. (1999). Defining lives: Occupation as identity: An essay on competence, coherence, and the creation of meaning, Eleanor Clarke Slagle lecture. *American Journal of Occupational Therapy, 53*, 547–558.

Clare, L. (2002). We'll fight it as long as we can: Coping with the onset of Alzheimer's. *Aging & Mental Health, 6*, 139–148.

Cooney, A. (2012). 'Finding home': A grounded theory on how older people 'find home' in long-term care settings. *International Journal of Older People Nursing, 7*, 188–199.

Cutchin, M. P. (2003). The process of mediated aging-in place: A theoretically and empirically based model. *Social Science and Medicine, 57*, 1077–1090.

Cutchin, M. P., Owen, S. V. & Chang, P. F. J. (2003). Becoming 'at home' in assisted living residences: Exploring place integration processes. *The Journals of Gerontology Series B: Psychological Sciences and Social Sciences, 58*(4), 234–243.

Cutchin, M. P. (2007). From society to self (and back) through place: Habit in transactional context. *OTJR: Occupation, Participation and Health, 27*(1 suppl), 50S–59S.

Cutchin, M. P. (2013). The complex process of becoming at-home in assisted living. In G. D. Rowles & M. Bernard (Eds.), *Environmental Gerontology: Making Meaningful Places in Old Age* (pp. 105–124). New York: Springer.

Dewey, J. (1957). *Human Nature and Conduct*. New York: Modern Library.

Greenwood, D., Loewenthal, D. & Rose, T. (2001). A relational approach to providing care for a person suffering from dementia. *Journal of Advanced Nursing, 36*(4), 583–590.

Haak, M. (2006). *Participation and interdependence in old age. Aspects of home and neighbourhood environment*. Lund: Department of Health Science, Division of Occupational Therapy and Gerontology, Lund University.

Hammell, K. W. (2004). Dimensions of meaning in the occupations of daily life. *Canadian Journal of Occupational Therapy, 71*, 296–305.

Harmer, B. J. & Orrell, M. (2008). What is meaningful activity for people with dementia living in care homes? A comparison of the views of older people with dementia, staff and family carers. *Aging & Mental Health, 12*, 548–558.

Hasselkus, B. R. (2002). *The Meaning of Everyday Occupation*. Thorofare, NJ: Slack.

Hayward, G. (1975). Home as an environmental and psychological concept. *Landscape, 20*(1), 2–9.

Jackson, J. (1996). Living a meaningful existence in old age. In R. Zemke & F. Clark (Eds.), *Occupational Science: The Evolving Discipline* (pp. 339–392). Philadelphia: F. A. Davis.

Kaufman, S. (1988). Illness, biography, and the interpretation of self following a stroke. *Journal of Aging Studies, 12,* 127–140.

Kielhofner, G. (Ed.) (2008). *Model of Human Occupation: Theory and Application.* Baltimore & Philadelphia: Lippincott Williams & Wilkins.

Kuo, A. (2011). A transactional view: Occupation as a means to create experiences that matter. *Journal of Occupational Science, 18,* 131–138.

Larson, E. A. & Zemke, R. (2003). Shaping the temporal patterns of our lives: The social coordination of occupation. *Journal of Occupational Science, 10*(2), 80–89.

Lee, V. S., Simpson, J. & Froggatt, K. (2013). A narrative exploration of older people's transitions into residential care. *Aging & Mental Health, 17,* 48–56.

Lemon, B. W., Bengtson, V. L. & Peterson, J. A. (1972). An exploration of the activity theory of aging: Activity types and life satisfaction among in-movers to a retirement community. *Journal of Gerontology, 27*(4), 511–523.

Lewin, F. A. (2001). The meaning of home among elderly immigrants: Directions for future research and theoretical development. *Housing Studies, 16,* 353–370.

Loboprabhu, S., Molinari, V. & Lomax, J. (2007). The transitional object in dementia: Clinical implications. *International Journal of Applied Psychoanalytic Studies, 4,* 144–169.

McColgan, G. (2005). A place to sit resistance strategies used to create privacy and home by people with dementia. *Journal of Contemporary Ethnography, 34,* 410–433.

de Medeiros, K., Rubinstein, R. & Doyle, P. (2013). A place of one's own: Reinterpreting the meaning of home among childless older women. In G. Rowles & M. Bernard (Eds.), *The Meaning of Home.* New York: Springer Publishing.

Milligan, C. (2012). *There's No Place Like Home: Place and Care in an Ageing Society.* Farnham: Ashgate Publishing, Ltd.

Narayanasamy, A. (2002). Spiritual coping mechanisms in chronically ill patients. *British Journal of Nursing, 11,* 1461–1470.

Oswald, F. & Wahl, H.-W. (2005). Dimensions of the meaning of home. In G. D. Rowles & H. Chaudhury (Eds.), *Home and Identity in Late Life: International Perspectives* (pp. 21–45). New York: Springer.

Rowles G. D. (1991). Beyond performance: Being in place as a component of occupational therapy. *American Journal of Occupational Therapy, 45*(3), 265–271.

Rowles, G. D. & Ravdal, H. (2002). Aging, place, and meaning in the face of changing circumstances. In R. S. Weiss & S. A. Bass (Eds.), *Challenges of the Third Age: Meaning and Purpose in Later Life.* (pp. 81–114). New York: Oxford University Press.

Rowles, G. D. (2003). The meaning of place as a component of self. In E. B. Crepeau, E. S. Cohn & B. A. Schell (Eds.), *Willard & Spackman's Occupational Therapy* (pp. 111–119). Philadelphia: Lippincott.

Rowles, G. D. (2008). Place in occupational science: A life course perspective on the role of environmental context in the quest for meaning. *Journal of Occupational Science, 15,* 127–135.

Seamon, D. (1980). Body-subject, time-space routines, and place-ballets. In A. Buttimer & D. Seamon, *The Human Experience of Space and Place* (pp. 148–165). Abingdon & New York: Routledge.

Schumaker, S. A. & Taylor, R. B. (1983). Toward a clarification of people place relationship: A model of attachment to place. In N. R. Feimer & E. S. Geller (Eds.), *Environmental Psychology: Direction and Perspectives*. New York: Praeger.

Shank, K. H. & Cutchin, M. P. (2010). Transactional occupations of older women aging-in-place: Negotiating change and meaning. *Journal of Occupational Science, 17*, 4–13.

Somerville, P. (1997). The social construction of home. *Journal of Architectural and Planning Research, 14*, 226–245.

Tanner, B., Tilse, C. & de Jonge, D. (2008). Restoring and sustaining home: The impact of home modifications on the meaning of home for older people. *Journal of Housing for the Elderly, 22*, 195–215.

Wenger, E. (1998). *Communities of Practice: Learning, Meaning, and Identity*. Cambridge: Cambridge University Press.

10

SELF-HELP, MUTUAL SUPPORT AND ADVOCACY: PEERS GETTING TOGETHER

Linda Örulv

Throughout history there have been many examples of groups of citizens organizing to give voice to their mutual concerns in public debate and to contribute to social change. That goes for everything from women's suffrage and the labor movement to LGBTQ[1] and disability rights. People join together in networks, communities, organisations and self-help groups for mutual support and exchange of experiences as well as advocacy and political activism.

This kind of self-organization is perhaps not regularly associated with people with dementia diseases; the notion of them being unaware of their life situation has proved to be surprisingly tenacious in spite of the growing research interest in early-stage perspectives and coping (Burgener & Berger, 2008). Recent research has shown that the awareness of people with dementia is commonly undervalued and that it is not determined solely by cognitive factors but depends on psychological and social factors as well (Clare et al., 2005). Furthermore, it is possible even for a person at late stages of dementia to reflect upon how one's life is affected by memory problems and other difficulties and how factors in the surroundings may help or make things worse (Clare et al., 2008b). It is time to realize that diagnosed citizens are not just passive recipients of other people's care but can and should be included in issues involving them (Bartlett & O'Connor, 2010; Naue & Kroll, 2008). This chapter has its point of departure in a piece of engaged research: I am probably the only researcher in the world who has followed a self-help group for people diagnosed with dementia diseases for as long as seven years, and I feel that I have a great responsibility to do their voice justice. I believe that we have only begun to recognize the experiences, perspectives and potential of people with dementia and that their getting together by their own initiative for self-help, mutual support and advocacy is an important, even necessary, way of achieving such recognition.

With earlier diagnoses it is now possible for people with dementia to have their voices heard like never before, in care planning and – not least – in public debate (Bartlett, 2014b; Beard, 2004b; Beard & Fox, 2008; Cayton, 2004; Mountain, 2006). Until now, elderly citizens have often been excluded from discussions on disability rights (Jönson & Taghizadeh Larsson, 2009). Although dementia is a disability according to the United Nations Convention on the

Rights of Persons with Disabilities, people with dementia diseases are still under-represented in disability studies (Bartlett, 2014b).[2] As late as 2012, Williamson (2012) argued for the need in the United Kingdom to apply the discourse about participation, empowerment, citizenship and social justice to people with dementia in the same way as it is applied to people with other long-term conditions. In several countries, like Sweden, policies and practices concerning disability do not even apply to people with dementia, unless they develop the disease before the age of 65. Instead this group of people falls under the umbrella of elderly care, where concepts like inclusion in the society have little place on the agenda, let alone the notion of disability rights (Taghizadeh Larsson, 2016). However, we may see a development with dementia diseases being regarded as cognitive disabilities that one may live with for a long time.

Interestingly, a self-help movement involving people with dementia is currently developing. This development is perhaps most prominent in Great Britain, where lately there has been a notable increase in the number of persons and groups engaging in dementia-related activism and mutual support (Williamson, 2012), especially in the Scottish Dementia Working Group (SDWG)[3] that devotes itself to influencing public policy and attitudes (Bartlett, 2014a, 2014b). However, a rising social movement for dementia is also manifesting itself on an international level in internet-based networks[4] (Clare et al., 2008a), in small local pioneering self-help groups (Örulv, 2011, 2012), in patient organisations that have started to engage advocates and council members with a diagnosis of their own (Beard, 2004a; McKillop et al., 2007), and in brave individuals taking it upon themselves to speak up about the barriers with which they have to struggle in everyday life (Knauss & Moyer, 2006; McKillop et al., 2007).

In self-help research it has been found that the organisation of groups and networks promotes interaction between the individual and the surrounding society and makes for a shift from a sufferer's position to that of an agent (Adamsen, 2002; Borkman, 1999). People with dementia diseases are no exception in this regard: participants in self-help groups and networks testify concerning the joy and meaning they find in helping others and contributing to raise public awareness. Central to these user-led organisations is the ambition to counteract stigmas associated with the diagnosis and work for more respectful treatment and recognition of their own voices and perspectives (Bartlett, 2014a; Clare et al, 2008a; Örulv, 2012). This chapter deals with that development – its driving forces and potential gains, the complexities of identity and diagnosis, the preconditions for self-management and organisation, the roles of professionals and the obstacles that still need to be challenged. The aim is to shed light on how, under the right circumstances, people with dementia diseases can unite and find the collective strength both to deal with their life challenges and to enter the public scene as agents of social change.

As an example adding to previous research, I will in the text occasionally return to a small Swedish self-help group, 'Ingrid's group', that I have been following for seven years. Ingrid's group has been around for a decade, with some of its original members still participating. The group started out as the initiative of a few enthusiasts with dementia diagnoses, Ingrid[5] being the ultimate driving force, and a dementia coordinator within the local municipal care. Group members have produced study material, arranged theme days, made statements in the media and given lectures to university students, care professionals, public authority staff and the public. Over the years the significance of the group as an arena for mutual support in early stages of the diseases has gradually received more recognition among local care practitioners and the social welfare board. In 2015 yet another group was started in the same municipality, as a municipal care initiative, with Ingrid's group as a raw model. Parallel to this process of receiving recognition, Ingrid's group has somehow lost its earlier air of grassroot activism and self-organised self-help and gradually turned into a regular support group with more of a professional agenda. As much as I am pleased with the fact that the need for an arena for getting together in the early stages has finally been officially recognised, I cannot but feel that something important has been lost.

Self-organising: driving-forces and potential gains

The activity of Ingrid's group started out as a dementia education planned and arranged by two women with dementia diagnoses and a coordinator who took a special interest in involving persons with dementia in their care planning. One of the women, Ingrid, on her own initiative had already gathered some of her neighbours for informal meetings on forgetfulness. She had also cooperated with the municipal care as an advisor, a lecturer and a mentor for others who had received a dementia diagnosis. Now she was eager to take part in this venture of planning an education addressing people with dementia, something that had not been available to her. Ingrid and the other woman played a major part as experts on living with a dementia disease and initiated the group discussions. The coordinator, a former nurse, contributed with her professional knowledge in accordance with the participants' wishes. Based on what had emerged as central issues in the discussion, themes for the following sessions were democratically decided. After these initial sessions, some participants agreed to both contribute to and take part in another round of sessions intended for new participants. This second group wished to continue meeting regularly after the education had ended, and they needed help with administration and location. It was decided that this was to be arranged within the local municipal care, and so 'Ingrid's group' was born.

The driving force behind Ingrid's group was for participants to be able to meet others in the same situation, learn about the condition and find coping strategies, but also to get people to talk about this feared condition and listen to the voices and perspectives of people living with the diagnosis. An important point of departure was that people with dementia were not just patients and passive recipients of care but agents in relation to their own condition and in relation to the society, both the welfare system and the public.

It has been suggested (Clare et al., 2008a) that self-help and mutual support networks could contribute to a more accepting and positive view of what it is like to live with dementia insofar as they empower people with dementia to play an active part in their care and treatment and to advocate for others to improve quality of life. For instance, members of the Dementia Advocacy and Support Network International (DASNI) expressed a feeling of collective strength and of being able to make valuable contributions to society. The sense of belonging, the feeling of being really understood and the culture of reciprocal support were key elements in this. Also, the network enabled information exchange and the development of accumulated experiential knowledge, similar to what has taken place in Ingrid's group (cf. Örulv, 2012). DASNI has reportedly given its members a purpose in life after the diagnosis, something to take pride in, and helped them to challenge stigma and regain a sense of control at least in some respects (Clare et al., 2008a). This corresponds with what Borkman (e.g. 1999) has reported with regard to self-help groups organized around a variety of problems that are shared by the members and dealt with actively in the context of voluntary and mutual engagement.

Advocacy can be part of the work that takes place in self-help groups and networks, but there are also transformational and coping processes going on as the participants learn, together, how to deal with their problems. Participants may or may not identify as activists. It is possible to engage in self-help and mutual support without being actively involved in advocacy, and vice versa, but there is a certain overlap. With or without advocacy work, what makes self-help and mutual support special is that it is based on the primary experience of the problem rather than some professional agenda. It develops because people recognize a challenge in their lives and get together to do something about it as agents (Borkman, 1999). With regard to dementia this means the development of a space that allows participants with dementia diseases to, on their own initiative, 'address and openly discuss dementia-related fears and concerns from their own perspective and in their own language' (Örulv, 2012, p. 13).

Not everyone will be interested in joining a self-help group or network or engaging in advocacy, just like not everyone is interested in joining organisations and associations (Borkman, 1999). Bartlett (2014a) has taken an interest in learning which mechanisms enable and motivate people with dementia to engage in dementia-related activism, either as part of a campaigning group or as an individual. She found that 'people with dementia are motivated to take action on behalf of the "cause" for three reasons: to protect self against further decline, to (re) gain respect and to create connections within the dementia community' (Bartlett, 2014a, p. 17).

Firstly, the participants in Bartlett's study (2014a) were well aware of their ongoing cognitive decline and adamant to do what they could while they were still able to do so. Taking action was seen as a way to slow the progress of the decline, or at least to do something constructive about it. Their subjective experience was that engaging in activism did make a difference to their personal health. Some participants reported that their engagements gave them a boost of energy or made them feel more alive. Others lived according to the motto 'use it or lose it', something that I recognise from Sinikka and Ingrid in 'Ingrid's group' as well. The latter is of course applicable to more than activism per se; Ingrid decided to maintain her mathematics skills and obtained some educational material and started practicing, and Sinikka kept using her computer in daily life because she noticed that she would otherwise forget how to use it. It is reasonable to assume that protecting self from further decline is a reason for people to engage in different forms of self-help, activism being one part of it.

Secondly, another important driving force for activism in Bartlett's (2014a) study was ending the oppression, in the shape of stigma and discrimination, and maintaining respect for oneself and for people with dementia diseases as a group, which is in line with what Clare and co-workers found (2008a). The participants felt that they were often seen as second-rate citizens or as imbeciles. Others talked down to them or above their heads. As a contrast, conferences and meetings in their campaigning enabled the participants to voice their concerns and to be recognised for their contribution (Bartlett, 2014a).

Thirdly, Bartlett (2014a) found that it was important to many of the participants, albeit not all of them, to be able to connect with other people with dementia. Getting organised was one way of doing this, as social networking was an integral part of activism. Most participants met others through meetings, conferences and other events. Some travelled far away to meet other activists, exchange ideas and bring those experiences back to their own group for inspiration. Getting together with other people with dementia was not only a means for activism, but also a matter of affinity or 'togetherness', learning from each other, sharing the experience and forming bonds, something that might foster solidarity.

Diagnosis and identity

One way or another, people with dementia coming together to engage in self-help, mutual support and advocacy need to find ways to deal with the fact that they have a dementia diagnosis and that it affects their social identity. It is certainly easier to organise and recruit members if people are willing, at least to some extent, to identify with their diagnosis and to meet and collaborate with others who share their diagnosis. This may be complicated by the fact that dementia has for a long time been associated with stigma or shame in various ways (Corner & Bond, 2004; Vernooij-Dassen et al., 2005) and may simply make people 'acutely uncomfortable' (Sterin, 2002, p. 8). Once a dementia diagnosis has been outed, stereotypical images often set boundaries to a person's identity and social life (Naue & Kroll, 2008; Sabat et al., 2004). Even well-meaning responses from family and friends may be overly protective and restrict one's autonomy more than necessary (MacQuarrie, 2005). Identifying with or being identified with the condition is thus social risk-taking. With that in mind it is understandable that early copers have often been found to downplay or deny their forgetfulness and other difficulties or use a number of compensating strategies to cover them up (e.g. Clare, 2002; van Dijkhuizen et al., 2006), or at least emphasise their remaining competences and active engagement (Offord et al., 2006). There seems to be a tangible need not to write oneself (at least one-sidedly) into a narrative of disease, passiveness and dependence.

On the other hand, the dementia diagnosis may also play a key role in coping with increasing difficulties. Beard and Fox (2008) found that support group participants (interviewed individually or in group) struggled to make sense of their situation, building on their everyday experiences as well as more technical jargon and biomedical frameworks. Diagnoses were sources both of oppression and of empowerment in this process, leading the authors to suggest an 'identity irony' in which individuals are robbed of their unique attributes while a group identity is solidified. The authors compare this to what has been described by others as a tension between agency and objectification (MacQuarrie, 2005) or hope and despair (Clare, 2002).

In the study by Beard and Fox (2008), the participants belonged to a professionally led support group rather than a self-help group, and the agenda was such that a medical lens was applied to the shared predicament. Yet, rather than being instantly relegated to a status of patient or impaired person, the participants negotiated their diagnosis by incorporating it. Normalisation efforts did not imply rejection of the diagnosis but rather an uneasy acceptance. Social interactions had to be managed so as to minimise social disenfranchisement. These respondents did not downplay, deny or cover up their difficulties but rather emphasised them. Their gain was a collective strength and a sense of camaraderie. 'Restorying' their lives as support group members, they reconstructed a new sense of self with different expectations. Disorderly experiences, shared by the group members, were normalised as part of accepting an illness identity, and at the same time the group afforded participants the opportunity to feel useful.

As Beard and Fox describe it, the participants were not passive recipients of their diagnoses, but employed interactional strategies in which the diagnosis was utilised as a resource to handle everyday matters and avoid restricting their lives more than necessary. In daily life, they were forced either to strategically navigate their identity, which demanded negotiations with others, or to accept a compromised identity. In relationships, they had to manage not only their symptoms but also the assumptions held by those with whom they were interacting (cf. Sabat et al., 2004). They had to vigilantly negotiate their everyday interactions and engage in constant impression management. Many found it beneficial to communicate their difficulties and need for assistance, as doing so granted both support and (ideally) empathy. This was also considered part of coming to terms with the disease. Moreover, it eased anxiety in awkward situations by justifying interactional breakdowns and the bending of social norms.

Dementia activists often bring their case forward by emphasising rather than downplaying the difficulties associated with the condition – by accentuating experiences and needs that are shared among the group members and affirmed in solidarity (Bartlett, 2014a). This was also the case with Ingrid's group for several years. In studying Ingrid's group at that point in time (Örulv, 2012), I found that the construction of a shared and more liberated perspective on life with dementia was a complex process that involved several subordinate processes. One dealt with how mutual experiential knowledge was put forward as a major source of authority, something that over time was complicated by the challenges posed by cognitive decline. Another process concerned dealing with the complex challenges of double stigmatisation, a two-front battle against both trivialisation of symptoms and dismissal due to stereotypical assumptions. A third process involved framing the identity as being interrelated with others and with society – as agents, depending on other agents, and as citizens.

Just like in the support group described by Beard and Fox (2008), the most active participants of Ingrid's group chose not to downplay, deny or cover up their difficulties, but rather to emphasise them and claim their right to support and understanding. In their advocacy work they took this further – negotiating everyday interactions was not the end of it, but they also made efforts to educate both professionals and the public based on their experiential knowledge of living with dementia diseases.

Yet, it was also clear that emphasising their difficulties was not done light-handedly and not without more agentive images being put forward as well. When presenting themselves in the group, some participants struggled hard to balance their increasing difficulties and support needs with their needs for control and a positive sense of self. These participants' self-presentations drew on rather contrasting storylines to give justice both to the despair felt when they were no longer able to cook without burning the pans or find their way out of the bedroom and to the social personae who were still able to sneak out late at night to play cards and have a drink with their friends without being noticed by their more puritan neighbors. When somebody positioned themselves one-sidedly in a negative way, other participants were quick to negotiate their story to remind them of their agency and their remaining competencies.

Preconditions for self-management and organisation

People with dementia have to a large extent 'been denied opportunities to regard themselves as agents in their own right', and this may become a downward spiral, characterised by learned helplessness, and therefore a self-fulfilling prophecy. Naue and Kroll suggest that concepts like learned resourcefulness be used to focus on people with dementia as agents capable of doing self-care rather than passive objects of other people's care (Naue & Kroll, 2008, p. 31). A development allowing for people with dementia diseases to be agentive with regard to their disease, and to organise and develop a voice of their own – as is the case with Ingrid's group, SDWG and DASNI – presupposes some basic elements. These elements could all contribute to learned resourcefulness.

First of all, a timely diagnosis is required so as to open up a window of opportunities, enabling the person to take action while still capable. Doctors may be hesitant to make a diagnosis because dementia diseases are feared and there is yet no cure available. Even if a diagnosis has been made, doctors' insecurity, paternalistic concerns and other factors have often interfered with the person's right to be informed of the diagnosis (Bamford et al., 2004; Gillies, 2000; for a review, see Werner et al., 2013). Being diagnosed with a dementia disease can certainly be an overwhelming and traumatic experience involving shock, grieving for losses, fear and frustration (Bryden, 2002; Clare et al., 2008a; Ostwald et al., 2002; Vernooij-Dassen et al., 2006). Information about the later stages of the disease might be painful to process; for the individual it may be difficult to find a balance where the information is useful and yet not too overwhelming (Clare, 2002). However, that does not mean that others have the right to withhold the information on their own authority.

According to a current research review (Werner et al., 2013), available studies indicate that most individuals with dementia diseases wish to be informed of their diagnosis and are able to deal with the information. In fact, Langdon and co-workers argue that the participants of their study, who had recently been diagnosed, were 'acutely sensitive to the responses of others to their diagnosis and well aware of strategies others adopt to protect them from the full impact of such a diagnosis'. They wished not to be protected from the truth about their condition but wanted clear, unambiguous and honest responses from people around them (Langdon et al., 2007, p. 999). As the SDWG-advocate Lynda Hogg puts it, 'people don't say openly what they think in case you might be upset. I'd rather be told why I can't do something. It doesn't help when people waffle to hide their reactions to a person with dementia' (McKillop et al., 2007, p. 15). Early diagnosis is one of the three most important campaigning priorities of SDWG, along with respite and medication (McKillop et al., 2007).

Fortunately, there are indications that attitudes in the medical profession have started to change with regard to the disclosure of dementia diagnosis, in favor of providing better information to the person diagnosed. Improvement of the doctor–patient communication in this process still needs to be addressed in training, especially when it comes to dealing with the still-remaining taboo surrounding the dementia diagnosis (Kaduszkievicz et al., 2008). Moniz-Cook and co-workers (2006) recommend pre-assessment (pre-diagnostic) psychosocial support in order to counter the fear associated with a dementia diagnosis and begin the process of enhancing self-management. More nuanced information and discussion could be part of this support, as well as information on how others have been able to maintain a good life with dementia. The media are full of frightening images of dementia, including scenarios of severe confusion and risky or socially demanding behaviors. These images are simplistic and only depict a fraction of how life with a dementia disease may evolve. They often overlook the potential of dealing with difficulties, making use of remaining resources and appreciating subjects for rejoicing that are still available in life. Instead of withholding sensitive information from the very person that it concerns the most, the information should be delivered in a context of support.

Access to information is essential; after all, knowledge is power. In addition to proper information about their diagnosis, there are many other kinds of information that people with dementia need in order to be able to stand up for their needs and rights. They need adequate information about the disease and which medical examinations and treatments are available. Furthermore, they need to know what forms of social and practical support are available and how to apply for them, which technical aids could be useful, how to manage their finances in the face of the evolving disease, etc. Traditionally, this information, if given at all, has mainly been addressed to the next of kin of persons with dementia, something that has been criticised by a number of researchers (Fitzsimmons & Buettner, 2003; Goldsilver & Gruneir, 2001; Mountain, 2006; Pearce et al., 2002; Örulv, 2012). Information to the next of kin has also been found to be insufficient, and critical voices have pointed out that elderly citizens have often been disregarded when it comes to patient education and follow-up procedures (Gillies, 2000; Visser, 2000).

Resourcefulness and agency need not be individual enterprises. On the contrary, self-help movements often operate according to the motto, 'You alone can do it, but you cannot do it alone' (Borkman, 1999). By getting together in self-help groups, organisations or networks, people with dementia diseases can support each other emotionally and practically throughout the challenges of daily life. Together they are stronger than alone. Also, together they can possibly develop a voice and make an impact on the public agenda. It is no coincidence that freedom of assembly has been so essential to the labor movement and other social movements. Lack of arenas for people with dementia to meet is a significant obstacle that is hopefully diminishing. The SDWG-advocate James McKillop, commenting on the lack of arenas before SDWG was established, asked, 'Could we not be trusted to have our own groups? What did they fear if people with dementia got together?' (McKillop et al., 2007). It is important that patient organisations address not only the next of kin, as is all too common even today, but also – or even especially – the diagnosed person. It is essential that people with dementia are not left to their own devices following a diagnosis, but have an infrastructure for getting in touch with others, if they wish to, and the support that they may require to be able to do so.

The 'to be or not to be' of professional facilitation

Ideally, self-help groups, networks and movements are self-organised. Yet when it comes to dementia diseases, there is often a lack of arenas for peers to get together, and therefore I believe that professionals could make a difference, in civil society or in community-based care. Because of the difficulties associated with dementia, professional facilitation may be useful and sometimes even required to start the activities and initiate the networking, and to manage practical arrangements (making reservations, managing budgets, making notes, managing contacts with authority persons that the participants wish to meet, etc.). This is sometimes the case in self-help organisations involving people without cognitive impairments as well, and it is not to be confused with having professionals set the agenda and actually lead the activities (Borkman, 1999). Professionals may also play an important part in helping individuals with dementia diseases to find each other, in the guise of dementia advisers who provide information and guidance to people with dementia and their families (Clarke et al., 2013; Keyes et al., 2014).

The existing literature addressing the issue of creating arenas for people with dementia diseases to come together for mutual support mainly deals with professionally led support groups. I would say that it suffers from overprotectiveness, a view that is shared by Clare and co-workers (2008a). Much of the literature is written from the perspective of care professionals and strongly emphasises the role of professional coordinators and the special difficulties of the participants. In one paper, it is suggested that facilitators be prepared at any time to adjust to fluctuations in the participants' mood, behavior, communication and cognition. Facilitators should then discreetly lead the participants back on the right track (Goldsilver & Gruneir, 2001). Other authors give advice, in a similar manner, on how to deal with participants' repetitions, communicative difficulties and agitation. The role of the professional facilitator is described as a complex balancing act of dealing with feelings of loss, fear and frustration together with the possibilities, remaining abilities and joy in the here and now (Yale & Snyder, 2002).

Apart from the fact that no actual empirical evidence is presented to support the alleged need for such extensive facilitation as described above, there are several potential problems to that assumption. First, there is an imminent risk that citizens with dementia diseases are left with very few meeting places if decision makers are convinced that professional supervision is always necessary, especially if advanced skills are required and if the coming together of people with dementia is depicted as a hazardous situation.

Second, this kind of professionally controlled agenda risks depriving the participants of their own agency. The example of Ingrid's group shows that citizens with early-stage dementia are able to find strategies for their problems together, without vigilant supervision from a facilitator ready to step in at any time to solve problems for them. Over the years I have found that most of the group members have been well aware of both their own and their peers' difficulties, and therefore communicative difficulties need not be such a big deal. Instead of masking their problems, participants have asked each other for help. They have also adjusted turn-taking to suit their own needs: the principle has been that when someone loses the thread, that person is allowed to hold the floor again as soon as he or she regains focus, without having to wait for his or her turn. Forgetfulness and other complications have been handled with empathy and smiles of recognition. In the absence of shame, there is no need for discreet balancing acts. Even when talking about difficult matters, the participants have been quite capable of dealing with their emotions and showing consideration for each other's difficulties.

A third aspect is that professionally led support groups may be too structured to support self-help, mutual support and advocacy. Research on self-help groups has shown that group processes change when self-government is replaced by external control. There is a decrease in engagement, solidarity and empathy and the participants tend to be more passive and less inclined to explore, share and expose themselves (Borkman, 1999; Jacobs & Goodman, 1989; Toro et al., 1988). Video recordings from a dementia support group showed that conversational topics were mainly controlled by the facilitators, even though the facilitators themselves thought that the participants were in charge. Nearly three-quarters of all interaction involved the facilitators, mostly with a single participant. Thus, there was little space for mutual support among the participants (Mason et al., 2005). Clare et al. (2008a) argue that the difficulties involved with dementia diseases need not warrant an increased need for professional facilitation but may in fact lead to an increased risk that professional facilitation of group conversations fosters passivity and dependence instead of encouraging agency.

That is *not* to say that professional support is redundant; it fills other needs than self-governed groups and networks. Overall, people with dementia often lack both arenas and opportunities for processing their feelings and coming to terms with their situation, both in connection with their diagnosis and later on (Goldsilver & Gruneir, 2001; Koppel & Dallos, 2007; Mountain, 2006; Naue & Kroll, 2008; Örulv, 2011, 2012; Vernooij-Dassen et al., 2006). Professionally led support groups could for instance provide tools for individuals in the moderate stage of the disease to position themselves in ways that support their self

(Hedman et al., 2014). Williamson (2012) points out that many groups that come together for peer support are grassroots and that participation may occur at all sorts of different levels depending on what people choose and are comfortable with. A citizenship movement should not be imposed on them, and a requirement that all groups should be led by people with dementia would be counterproductive.

Clare and coworkers (2008a, p. 10) maintain that there is indeed a role for professional facilitation, but it is important to also 'consider the possibility that people with early-stage dementia can organize themselves and engage in self-help and mutual support under certain circumstances without professional facilitation, and that for some individuals this may bring even greater benefits'. The contribution and competency of the participants should not be underestimated, and their agency should not be removed. Together they can take a great responsibility for the agenda and for the development of their group, network or organisation. With the right support, people with dementia, especially in the earlier stages, are able to form and run their own groups if they wish to do so (McKillop et al., 2007).

Obstacles for self-advocacy

When it comes to advocacy, according to Bartlett, people with dementia diseases are habitually reduced to patients and to passive recipients of welfare while their potentialities as citizens and as agents are denied. They have to grapple not only with their impairment but also with attitudinal barriers, as if the former was not enough (Bartlett, 2014b). These barriers include negative public perceptions of dementia and ageism (Beard, 2004a).

As an example, the advocates Knauss and Moyer (2006) describe the frustration of having stories to tell from an insider's perspective, for instance about the values of early diagnosis, but not the opportunities and resources to do so. Furthermore, they problematise the fact that in research people with dementia are often treated as 'objects to be "randomized" and "evaluated" to provide "data" rather than being treated as people who can provide wisdom' (Knauss & Moyer, 2006, p. 71). They are not recognised for the contribution that they can make based both on their primary experience of the disease and on the variety of competencies that they may possess that are still intact. For instance, studies of assistive technology would benefit from the knowledge of technical experts who have themselves been diagnosed with dementia (Knauss & Moyer, 2006). After all, as Bartlett (2014b, p. 1293) puts it, 'people with dementia are not a homogenous group of "passive patients" but a diverse group of men and women with a range of resources to draw upon'.

Historically, people with dementia have depended on others to talk on their behalf because of their marginalised situation. As Beard puts it (2004a, p. 797), '[c]ompared with the health social movements of other diseases, the Alzheimer's disease movement has been slow in identifying and implementing public spokespersons'. Traditionally, family members or other loved ones have been the spokespersons, and attempts to give voice to people with Alzheimer's disease from their own perspectives have encountered barriers. People with dementia have often been assumed unable or unwilling to talk about their situation, or even too vulnerable to approach, wherefore others have taken on themselves the role of speaking for people with dementia. Unfortunately, the lack of spokespersons with the condition contributes to maintaining the negative image of people with dementia as incompetent or confused – something that makes it even harder to speak up; it is a downward spiral (Beard, 2004a).

Persons with dementia diseases who do speak up are often met with disbelief because of stereotypical assumptions: if they are able to engage in public debate and assert themselves like that, or in other ways present themselves as capable, then they cannot possibly have a dementia disease (Bartlett, 2014b; Clare at al., 2008a; O'Connor et al., 2010; Örulv, 2012). Bartlett (2014b, p. 1300) describes this phenomenon as 'oppression linked to normative expectations about what someone with dementia "should" be like'.

Even today, people with dementia are often treated paternalistically to protect them from having to deal with public perceptions and stigma or more generally from public humiliation or challenging situations (Beard, 2004a). This was the case for Ingrid in her early engagements, before the self-help group had started. In 2005, she gave a much-appreciated talk at a national workshop on dementia care together with the local dementia nurse and district nurse. Her participation was almost stopped by the local head of primary health care who, according to interviews with Ingrid and the dementia nurse, said that this was the most irresponsible thing she had ever heard of. Ingrid had to get her physician to attest that she was well enough to take part in the workshop.

While the condition of elderly persons with dementia seems to be such a cause for concern that their engagement in advocacy may be prohibited, paradoxically enough it is often at the same time remarkably trivialised. For some reason people often assume that it is not such a big deal for an older person to have memory problems (cf. the trivialisation of symptoms as experienced by the participants of Ingrid's group). In her study of the Alzheimer's disease movement, Beard found that the elderly spokespersons were therefore not taken seriously (Beard, 2004a). People with early-onset diseases made more effective spokespersons in that sense, but they are less common and their disease progression is more rapid, which makes it hard for them to take on the role. Earlier diagnoses make it possible for people with the condition to engage in public discourse, but diagnostics are still uncertain and doctors, according to associate responders, tend to be avoidant, as problematised above. Even when diagnoses are made (and properly communicated), doctors do not refer people to the association quickly enough (Beard, 2004a). The timing may be critical; according to Bartlett

(2014a), a window of possibilities opens up just as the person has processed the initial shock and settled into the illness. At that time the person might value the possibility to engage in collective action, wherefore it is problematic that individualised care and support is often the only thing that is offered.

Bartlett (2014b) points out that it is important to address to what extent people who campaign for social change are hurt by negative stereotypes and stigma surrounding dementia and what are the personal costs of coming out. Any oppressive practices need to be identified and avoided.

Internal obstacles for self-advocacy within the dementia movement

Some of the oppressing practices have developed within the dementia movement itself. The Alzheimer's Association, a strong force behind the movement in the United States, was established by care providers and scientists and therefore strongly committed to certain goals: research on causes and cures, caregivers' situations and long-term care. Diagnostic advancements have made it possible for people with the condition to join the movement, and their previously unheard perspectives can now be incorporated and their different needs and concerns put on the agenda. However, that means competition for resources as well as rival ideologies – between the biomedical perspective and the variety of subjective experiences, between cure and quality of life (Beard, 2004a).

Despite the best of intentions, Beard found that there were a number of competing organisational needs that conflicted with the objective of incorporating perspectives of people with dementia into planning care, services and policies. Some obstacles were due to internal dynamics, including organisational habits, organisational survival and organisational structure. The force of habit is strong, and the long tradition of working with family support and allocation of resources for biomedical research may hinder the inclusion of people with dementia. When it comes to survival as a voluntary organisation, relying on private donations, the association has not always chosen to portray people with dementia in a favorable way. Cynically enough, positive images of people with the condition are not effective tools for fund-raising, whereas devastating victim images are. Also, donors tend to earmark their funding for certain objectives, regardless of what the association staff thinks, which makes it difficult to develop and implement new objectives. The decentralised organisational structure makes it hard for new perspectives to have an impact on a larger scale (Beard, 2004).

Furthermore, investing in spokespersons with progressive diseases can be seen as riskier, as their window of time is smaller – although according to Bartlett (2014a) the sense of elapsing time can also be a driving force for activism. From the point of view of the organisation, the investment pays out for a shorter time period. Also, it may be more difficult to plan speaking engagements because it is difficult to predict how the person will feel on a particular day. In that sense, spokespersons with dementia diagnoses are perceived as less effective (Beard, 2004a). On the other hand, the targeted audience is often people who are in different ways responsible for dementia care. One might argue that, as the coordinators of Ingrid's group have pointed out, if these people are not patient enough to be lenient with fluctuations in the abilities of people with dementia, then perhaps they should not be responsible for dementia care in the first place.

Sometimes the process of campaigning as a dementia self-advocate involves experiences of being taken advantage of as an alibi in an oppressive system (Bartlett, 2014b) – or as Knauss and Moyer (2006) puts it, as a 'sideshow attraction' – or used as an unpaid resource, although not receiving payment can also mean avoiding a position of dependence. Sometimes it is unrewarding when professionals do not see what effort it takes because of the dementia disease or what costs are paid in terms of exhaustion. There may also be emotional consequences that go unseen in public, as campaigning can be draining and even hurtful, sometimes in the shape of something similar to survivor's guilt that results in the person feeling ashamed for not being more impaired. Giving lectures may involve terror of forgetting things. Social conventions may be demanding because of the cognitive changes. A sense of duty may pressure the person to perform even if he or she does not feel up to it. Practical problems add to the burden, for instance when campaigners forget to claim expenses or struggle with administrative processes. Some participants reported that they regretted their loss of anonymity due to campaign work. Getting involved can be empowering, but in the case of dementia, as in several other forms of disability, there is also a high price to pay – especially when support needs are not met (Bartlett, 2014b).

Given that high price, the protectiveness of people with dementia when it comes to advocacy is perhaps understandable. Not everyone may be willing or able to participate, and that is important to be aware of. On the other hand, for those who are genuinely committed to it, it is important to support and allow them the opportunity. As Beard (2004b, p. 426) puts it: 'Bringing the voice of previously marginalized people to the forefront dispels myths of inability, unwillingness, or lack of desire to express subjective experiences.' There is an imperative need for development of rules for campaigning that allow people with dementia diseases to be themselves. The social rules that participants feel they have to abide by are all too often created by non-impaired people, and user-led organisations can make a change in this respect (Bartlett, 2014b).

Discussion

Not very long ago it was generally assumed that dementia diseases would make it impossible for people to advocate for themselves and to organise. Clearly this is not the case. Dementia diseases affect a person's cognitive abilities and communication with others to a varying degree, but the diseases per se may not necessarily prevent a person from organising in groups, networks or patient organisations (Bartlett, 2014a, 2014b; Beard, 2004a). Ingrid's group illustrates this clearly, along with the Scottish Dementia Working Group and the Dementia Advocacy and Support Network International. The body of research shows that there are many driving forces behind the rising dementia self-help movement. Getting together with peers involves a sense of belonging and of being genuinely understood and an opportunity to share experiences and learn from each other. Mutual support means being able not only to receive something from others but also to make a contribution. It means being agentive. The perspectives that develop in self-organised groups and networks challenge stigma and negative expectations and paint a more nuanced and constructive picture of what it is like to live with a dementia disease. When participants speak up and voice these perspectives, they are not only developing coping strategies but also fighting against oppression, as agents of social change (Bartlett, 2014a; Clare et al., 2008a; Örulv, 2012).

In order to facilitate this development, it is important that we recognise people with dementia diseases for the agency and the resources that they do possess, and at the same time recognise their need for support. There should be no contradiction in taking people's difficulties seriously and accommodating them while at the same time appreciating that these persons may have an agenda of their own and have a great deal to offer. There is a fine line between being supportive and being paternalistically overprotective, and that line needs to be carefully observed and respected. Alongside care and support, people with dementia need access to their diagnosis, to information and to arenas. They need the infrastructures necessary to connect with others and the space to develop their own strategies, agendas and voices. In advocacy they need to be able to be involved on their own terms rather than having to play by healthy people's rules. Care professionals, family members and other healthy people who are engaged in dementia advocacy need to find ways to be allies rather than compete for resources and influence.

It is imperative to find ways of putting dementia on the public agenda without resorting to using horrifying images as a means to allocate resources, as these images reduce people with dementia to tragic cases, undermine their agency and deprive them of a voice of their own. As long as dementia is seen as these worst-case scenarios, 'coming out' as diagnosed is not only psychologically demanding but also social risk taking. Therefore, many people may refrain from identifying with the diagnosis and seeking support, let alone organising and doing campaign work. Today people with dementia diseases often lack venues for meeting others in their situation and their voices are rarely heard in public debate. That is highly problematic. However, creating the opportunities will probably not solve the problem as if by a stroke of magic. It may take a while for many people with dementia to become comfortable with the idea of identifying with their disease enough to join a movement, find collective strength and develop a shared voice. Nuancing the image of dementia and overcoming stereotypes that set boundaries to people is a long-term process that requires patience. Both commitment and financial resources are needed to develop new arenas and support the existing ones (Clarke et al., 2013; Williamson, 2012). The pioneers of this growing movement play an important part – self-advocates and enthusiasts who build networks to accomplish something together. Not everyone will be able or willing to shoulder that burden, and we need to respect this, while at the same time working hard to remove the obstacles for and enable those who are prepared to make a difference. The more pioneers leading the way, the easier it will be for others to follow.

Notes

1   Lesbian, gay, bisexual, transgender, and questioning/queer.
2   The inclusion of people with dementia and of dementia research and dementia advocacy organizations in the 2015 International Conference 'Claiming Full Citizenship: Self Determination, Personalization, Individualized Funding' in Vancouver was, however, an important milestone in this respect.
3   An activist network run by people with dementia and founded in 2001 – see www.sdwg.org.uk/videos/home/history-of-sdwg/, accessed 3 December 2015.
4   The Dementia Advocacy and Support Network International (DASNI) started in 2000 – see www.dasninternational.org/2003/history.php, accessed 3 December, 2015.
5   A pseudonym used according to the ethical standards for research in Sweden, although the individual herself has chosen to come forward with her real name in the media in order to reduce the shame surrounding dementia diagnoses.

References

Adamsen, L. (2002). 'From victim to agent': The clinical and social significance of self-help group participation for people with life-threatening diseases. *Scandinavian Journal of Caring Sciences, 16*, 224–231.
Bamford, C., Lamont, S., Eccles, M., Robinson, L., May, C. & Bond, J. (2004). Disclosing a diagnosis of dementia: A systematic review. *International Journal of Geriatric Psychiatry, 19*, 151–169.

Bartlett, R. (2014a). The emergent modes of dementia activism. *Ageing & Society, 34,* 623–644.

Bartlett, R. (2014b). Citizenship in action: The lived experiences of citizens with dementia who campaign for social change. *Disability & Society, 29,* 1291–1304.

Bartlett, R. & O'Connor, D. (2010). *Broadening the Dementia Debate: Towards Social Citizenship.* Bristol: Policy Press.

Beard, R. L. (2004a). Advocating voice: Organizational, historical and social milieu of the Alzheimer's disease movement. *Sociology of Health & Illness, 26,* 797–819.

Beard, R. L. (2004b). In their voices: Identity preservation and experiences of Alzheimer's disease. *Journal of Aging Studies, 18,* 415–428.

Beard, R. L. & Fox, P. J. (2008). Resisting social disenfranchisement: Negotiating collective identities and everyday life with memory loss. *Social Science & Medicine, 66,* 1509–1520.

Borkman, T. (1999). *Understanding Self-Help/Mutual Aid: Experiential Learning in the Commons.* New Brunswick, NJ & London: Rutgers University Press.

Bryden (Boden), C. (2002). A person-centred approach to counselling, psychotherapy and rehabilitation of people diagnosed with dementia in the early stages. *Dementia: The International Journal of Social Research and Practice, 1,* 141–156.

Burgener, S. C. & Berger, B. (2008). Measuring perceived stigma in persons with progressive neurological disease: Alzheimer's dementia and Parkinson's disease. *Dementia: The International Journal of Social Research and Practice, 7,* 31–53.

Cayton, H. (2004). Telling stories: Choices and challenges on the journey of dementia. *Dementia: The International Journal of Social Research and Practice, 3,* 9–17.

Clare, L. (2002). We'll fight as long as we can: Coping with the onset of Alzheimer's disease. *Ageing & Mental Health, 6,* 139–148.

Clare, L., Roth, I. & Pratt, R. (2005). Perceptions of change over time in early-stage Alzheimer's disease: Implications for understanding awareness and coping style. *Dementia: The International Journal of Social Research and Practice, 4,* 487–520.

Clare, L., Rowlands, J. M. & Quin, R. (2008a). Collective strength: The impact of developing a shared social identity in early-stage dementia. *Dementia: The International Journal of Social Research and Practice, 7,* 9–30.

Clare, L., Rowlands, J., Bruce, E., Surr, C. & Downs, M. (2008b). 'I don't do like I used to': A grounded theory approach to conceptualizing awareness in people with moderate to severe dementia living in long-term care. *Social Science & Medicine, 66,* 2366–2377.

Clarke, C., Keyes, S., Wilkinson, H. & Alexjuk, J. (2013). *Healthbridge: The National Evaluation of Peer Support Networks and Dementia Advisers in implementation of the National Dementia Strategy for England.* In a Department of Health Policy Research Programme Project. Department of Health.

Corner, L. & Bond, J. (2004). Being at risk of dementia: Fears and anxieties of older adults. *Journal of Aging Studies, 18,* 143–155.

van Dijkhuizen, M., Clare, L. & Pearce, A. (2006). Striving for connection. Appraisal and coping among women with early-stage Alzheimer's disease. *Dementia: The International Journal of Social Research and Practice, 5,* 73–94.

Fitzsimmons, S. & Buettner, L. L. (2003). Health promotion for the mind, body and spirit: A college course for older adults with dementia. *American Journal of Alzheimer's Disease and Other Dementias, 18,* 282–290.

Gillies, B. A. (2000). A memory like clockwork: Accounts of living through dementia. *Aging & Mental Health, 4,* 366–374.

Goldsilver, P. M. & Gruneir, M. R. B. (2001). Early stage dementia group: An innovative model of support for individuals in the early stages of dementia. *American Journal of Alzheimer's Disease and Other Dementias, 16*, 109–114.

Hedman, R., Hellström, I., Ternestedt, B. M., Hansebo, G. & Norberg, A. (2014). Social positioning by people with Alzheimer's disease in a support group. *Journal of Aging Studies, 28*, 11–21.

Jacobs, M. K. & Goodman, G. (1989). Psychology and self-help groups: Predictions on a partnership. *American Psychologist, 44*, 536–545.

Jönson, H. & Taghizadeh Larsson, A. (2009). The exclusion of older people in disability activism and policies – a case of inadvertent ageism? *Journal of Aging Studies, 23*, 69–77.

Kaduszkievicz, H., Bachmann, C. & van den Bussche, H. (2008). Telling 'the truth' in dementia – Do attitude and approach of general practitioners and specialists differ? *Patient Education and Counseling, 70*, 220–226.

Keyes, S., Clarke, C., Wilkinson, H., Alexjuk, J., Wilcockson, J., Robinson, L., Reynolds, J., McClelland, S., Corner, L. & Cattan, M. (2014). 'We're all thrown in the same boat...': A qualitative analysis of peer support in dementia care. *Dementia: The International Journal of Social Research and Practice, 0*(0), 1–18. doi:10.1177/1471301214529575.

Knauss, J. & Moyer, D. (2006). The role of advocacy in our adventure with Alzheimer's. *Dementia: The International Journal of Social Research and Practice, 5*, 67–72.

Koppel, O. S. B. & Dallos, R. (2007). The development of memory difficulties: A journey into the unknown. *Dementia: The International Journal of Social Research and Practice, 6*, 193–213.

Langdon, S. A., Eagle, A. & Warner, J. (2007). Making sense of dementia in the social world: A qualitative study. *Social Science & Medicine, 64*, 989–1000.

MacQuarrie, C. R. (2005). Experiences in early stage Alzheimer's disease: Understanding the paradox of acceptance and denial. *Aging & Mental Health, 9*, 430–441.

Mason, E., Clare, L. & Pistrang, N. (2005). Processes and experiences of mutual support in professionally-led support groups for people with early-stage dementia. *Dementia: The International Journal of Social Research and Practice, 4*, 87–112.

McKillop, J., Hogg, L. & Houston, A. (2007). Having dementia, being a citizen. *The Journal of Dementia Care*, July/August, 14–15.

Moniz-Cook, E., Manthorpe, J., Carr, I., Gibson, G. & Vernooij-Dassen, M. (2006). Facing the future: A qualitative study of older people referred to a memory clinic prior to assessment and diagnosis. *Dementia: The International Journal of Social Research and Practice, 5*, 375–395.

Mountain, G. (2006). Self-management for people with early dementia: An exploration of concepts and supporting evidence. *Dementia: The International Journal of Social Research and Practice, 5*, 429–446.

Naue, U. & Kroll, T. (2008). 'The demented other': Identity and difference in dementia. *Nursing Philosophy, 10*, 26–33.

O'Connor, D., Phinney, A. & Hulko, W. (2010). Dementia at the intersections: A unique case study exploring social location. *Journal of Aging Studies, 24*, 30–39.

Offord, R. E., Hardy, G., Lamers, C. & Bergin, L. (2006). Teaching, teasing, flirting and fighting: A study of interactions between participants in a psychotherapeutic group for people with a dementia syndrome. *Dementia: The International Journal of Social Research and Practice, 5*, 167–195.

Örulv, L. (2011). Demens: diagnosen som utmanar våra rädslor och fördomar. In G. Drakos & L. C. Hydén (Eds.), *Diagnos & identitet* (pp. 100–129). Stockholm: Gothia förlag.

Örulv, L. (2012). Reframing dementia in Swedish self-help group conversations: Constructing citizenship. *The International Journal of Self-help and Self-care, 6*, 9–41.

Ostwald, S. K., Duggleby, W. & Hepburn, K. W. (2002). The stress of dementia: View from the inside. *American Journal of Alzheimer's Disease and Other Dementias, 17*, 303–312.

Pearce, A., Clare, L. & Pistrang, N. (2002). Managing sense of self: Coping in the early stages of Alzheimer's disease. *Dementia: The International Journal of Social Research and Practice, 1*, 173–192.

Sabat, S. R., Napolitano, L. & Fath, H. (2004). Barriers to the construction of a valued social identity: A case study of Alzheimer's disease. *American Journal of Alzheimer's Disease and Other Dementias, 19*, 177–185.

Sterin, G. J. (2002). Essay on a word: A lived experience of Alzheimer's disease. *Dementia: The International Journal of Social Research and Practice, 1*, 7–10.

Taghizadeh Larsson, A. (2016). Funktion. In S. Johansson & A. Taghizadeh Larsson (Eds.), *Förändringsperspektiv på äldreomsorg – att leva som andra* (pp. 73–89). Malmö: Gleerups.

Toro, P. A., Reischl, T. M., Zimmerman, M. A., Rappaport, J., Seidman, E., Luke, D. A. & Roberts, L. J. (1988). Professionals in mutual help groups: Impact on social climate and members' behavior. *Journal of Consulting and Clinical Psychology, 56*, 631–632.

Vernooij-Dassen, M., Derksens, E., Scheltens, P. & Moniz-Cook, E. (2006). Receiving a diagnosis of dementia: The experience over time. *Dementia: The International Journal of Social Research and Practice, 5*, 397–410.

Vernooij-Dassen, M., Moniz-Cook, E., Woods, R., De Lepeleire, J., Leuschner, A., Zanetti, O., De Rotrou, J., Kenny, G., Franco, M., Peters, V. & Iliffe, S. (2005). Factors affecting timely recognition and diagnosis of dementia across Europe: From awareness to stigma. *International Journal of Geriatric Psychiatry, 20*, 377–386.

Visser, A. (2000). Chronic diseases, aging, and dementia: Implications for patient education and counseling. *Patient Education and Counseling, 39*, 293–309.

Werner, P., Karnieli-Miller, O. & Eidelman, S. (2013). Current knowledge and future directions about the disclosure of dementia: A systematic review of the first decade of the 21st century. *Alzheimer's & Dementia, 9*, e74–e88.

Williamson, T. (2012). A stronger collective voice for people with dementia. Joseph Rowntree Foundation, York, UK. Available to download from www.jrf.org.uk/publications/stronger-collective-voice, accessed 13 December 2016.

Yale, R. & Snyder, L. (2002). The experience of support groups for persons with early-stage Alzheimer's disease and their families. In P. B. Harris (Ed.), *The Person with Alzheimer's Disease: Pathways to Understanding the Experience* (pp. 228–245). Baltimore, MD & London: Johns Hopkins University Press.

INDEX

Printed by Printforce, the Netherlands